U.S. Department of Homeland Security

United States Coast Guard

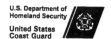

Commandant
United States Coast Guard

2100 Second Street, S.W.
Washington, DC 20593-0001
Staff Symbol: G-RPP
Phone: (202) 267-0518
Fax: (202) 267-4085
Email: ctantillo@comdt.uscg.mil

COMDTPUB P3120.17A

AUG 1 8 2006

COMMANDANT PUBLICATION P3120.17A

Subj: U.S. COAST GUARD INCIDENT MANAGEMENT HANDBOOK

Ref: (a) Homeland Security Presidential Directive Five (HSPD-5)
        (b) National Incident Management System (NIMS), March 2004
        (c) National Response Plan (NRP), December 2005
        (d) Coast Guard NIMS-NRP Implementation Plan, Dec 2004
        (e) Alignment with the National Incident Management System and National Response Plan, COMDTINST 16000.27 (series)
        (f) Incident Command System, COMDTINST 3120.14 (series)
        (g) Coast Guard Incident Command System Implementation Plan, COMDTINST M3120.15 (series)

1. <u>PURPOSE</u>. The Coast Guard Incident Management Handbook (IMH) is designed to assist Coast Guard personnel in the use of the National Incident Management System (NIMS) Incident Command System (ICS) during multi-contingency response operations and pla~~~~ Incident Management Handbook is an easy reference job aid for responders. document, but rather guidance for response personnel.

2. <u>ACTION</u>. Area, district, maintenance and logistics commanders, commandir headquarters units, assistant commandants for directorates, and commanding Guard units should disseminate this as widely as possible to all Coast Guard p response operations.

3. <u>DIRECTIVES AFFECTED</u>. U.S. Coast Guard Incident Management Handbo P3120.17, dated April 11, 2001 is cancelled.

4. <u>BACKGROUND</u>.

DISTRIBUTION – SDL No. 145

	a	b	c	d	e	f	g	h	i	j	k	l	m	n	o	p	q	r	s	t
A																				
B	500	750	750		525									*						
C	25				50									50		25				
D		500		50																
E																				
F																				
G																				
H																				

NON-STANDARD DISTRIBUTION: B:n 1500 copies

a. The Homeland Security Act of 2002 and Homeland Security Presidential Directive Five (HSPD-5), "Management of Domestic Incidents," fundamentally changed how the U.S. prepares for and responds to domestic incidents. As the primary documents for implementing HSPD-5, the NIMS and the National Response Plan (NRP) established a comprehensive approach to incident management and instituted a new national policy and procedures for response. The NIMS ICS is a standardized, all hazard – all risk approach to managing crisis response operations as well as non-crisis events whose principles can be applied to all types of incidents. The Department of Homeland Security (DHS) required all Federal departments and agencies to adopt and fully implement the NIMS ICS by September 2005 as outlined in references (a) through (d).

b. The IMH was revised to include information related to references (a) through (e) as well as small improvements and new tools for the user. The IMH is organized so that the generic information applicable to all types of responses is at the front of the document. For example, the duties and responsibilities of a Planning Section Chief are found in the generic planning section chapter since a Planning Section Chief's job description under ICS does not change from one type of incident to another. The remainder of the IMH is divided into supplements tailored to eight types of incidents the Coast Guard is likely to respond: Terrorism, Search and Rescue; Law Enforcement; Oil Spills; Hazardous Substance Releases (chemical, biological, radiological, and nuclear); Marine Fire; Multi-Casualty and Incidents of National Significance under the NRP.

5. JOB AID AVAILABILITY. USCG NIMS ICS job aids noted in the Handbook and can be found on the Internet at http://homeport.uscg.mil. Coast Guard training courses, if needed, will incorporate the USCG NIMS ICS standard forms since they can be used for the full range of contingencies.

6. FORMS AVAILABILITY. USCG NIMS ICS standard forms included in the Handbook and can be found on the Internet at http://homeport.uscg.mil. Coast Guard training courses, if needed, will incorporate the USCG NIMS ICS standard forms since they can be used for the full range of contingencies.

WAYNE E. JUSTICE
Rear Admiral, U.S. Coast Guard
Director of Enforcement and Incident Management

For sale by the Superintendent of Documents, U.S. Government Printing Office
Internet: bookstore.gpo.gov Phone: toll free (866) 512-1800; DC area (202) 512-1800
Fax: (202) 512-2104 Mail: Stop IDCC, Washington, DC 20402-0001

ISBN 978-0-16-077139-2

U.S. COAST GUARD
INCIDENT MANAGEMENT HANDBOOK

INCIDENT COMMAND SYSTEM
(ICS)

PREPARED BY U.S. COAST GUARD
WASHINGTON, D.C. 20593

2006 EDITION

Comments
Please provide comments on this manual to
the Coast Guard Headquarters Office of
Response, Incident Management and
Preparedness:

USCG Commandant (G-RPP)
2100 Second Street, S.W.
Washington, D.C. 20593-0001

For sale by the
U S Government Printing Office
Superintendent of Documents
732 North Capitol St. NW
Washington, DC 20401
Phone: 202-512-0000
Http://www.gpo.gov
Online bookstore: http://bookstore.gpo.gov/

TABLE OF CONTENTS

THIS PAGE INTENTIONALLY LEFT BLANK

TABLE OF CONTENTS **TABLE OF CONTENTS**

CHAPTER 1

INTRODUCTION

The U.S. Coast Guard Incident Management Handbook (IMH) is designed to assist Coast Guard personnel in the use of the National Incident Management System (NIMS) Incident Command System (ICS) during response operations. The IMH is intended to be used as an easy reference job aid for responders. It is not a policy document, but rather guidance for response personnel. During development of the IMH, it was recognized that eighty-percent of all response operations share common principles, procedures and processes. The other twenty-percent of response operations are unique to the type of incident, such as a search and rescue case or an oil spill. The handbook is laid out so that the generic information applicable to all responses is presented up-front. For example, the duties and responsibilities of the Planning Section Chief (PSC) are found in the generic section since a PSC's job description under ICS does not change from one type of incident to another. The remainder of the IMH is divided into eight types of incidents the Coast Guard is most likely to respond to. They are:

Terrorism
Search and Rescue
Law Enforcement
Oil Spills
Hazardous Substance (Chemical, Biological,
    Radiological, Nuclear)
Marine Fire Fighting and Salvage
Event Management and National Special Security
    Event (NSSE)
Multi-Casualty

Each of the scenario chapters pertain to a specific type of incident provides a situation from which to illustrate how an incident starts off with first responders and escalates to a large multi-agency response organization. The organizational charts in each chapter are only intended as **examples** of how an ICS organization may be developed to respond to that type of incident. Additionally, in each chapter are incident-specific job descriptions that have proven valuable in past response operations. An example of an incident-specific position would be the Vessel Disposition Group Supervisor located in the Law Enforcement chapter.

Coast Guard response personnel may come from any component of the Coast Guard (Active Duty, Reserve, Auxiliary, or Civilian Employees). Responders should have a basic understanding of NIMS and NIMS ICS to ensure they can effectively operate within the ICS organization and properly use and understand this IMH. Please note that acronyms are used extensively throughout this handbook and will not necessarily be identified when first used, however, an acronym list can be found in chapter 25.

CHAPTER 2

COMMON RESPONSIBILITIES

COMMON RESPONSIBILITIES

The following checklist is applicable to all personnel in an ICS organization:

a. Receive assignment from your agency, including:
- Job assignment (e.g. designation, position, etc.).
- Brief overview of type and magnitude of incident.
- Resource order number and request number/Travel Orders (TONO).
- Travel instructions including reporting location and reporting time.
- Any special communications instructions (e.g. travel, radio frequency).
- Monitor incident related information from media, internet, etc., if available.
- Assess personal equipment readiness for specific incident and climate (e.g. medications, money, computer, medical record, etc.). Maintain a checklist of items and possibly a personal Go-Kit.
- Inform others as to where you are going and how to contact you.
- Review Coast Guard Incident Management Handbook.
- Take advantage of available travel to rest prior to arrival.

b. Upon arrival at the incident, check in at the designated check-in location. Check-in may be found at any of the following locations:
- Incident Command Post (ICP).
- Base.
- Staging Areas.

- Helibases.

Note: If you are instructed to report directly to an on-scene assignment, check in with the Division/Group Supervisor or the Operations Section Chief.

c. Receive briefing from immediate supervisor.

d. Agency representatives from assisting or cooperating agencies report to the Liaison Officer (LNO) at the ICP after check-in.

e. Acquire work materials.

f. Abide by organizational code of ethics.

g. Participate in IMT meetings and briefings as appropriate.

h. Ensure compliance with all safety practices and procedures. Report unsafe conditions to the Safety Officer.

i. Supervisors shall maintain accountability for their assigned personnel with regard as to exact location(s), personal safety, and welfare at all times, especially when working in or around incident operations.

j. Organize and brief subordinates.

k. Know your assigned communication methods and procedures for your area of responsibility and ensure that communication equipment is operating properly.

l. Use clear text and ICS terminology (no codes) in all radio communications.

m. Complete forms and reports required of the assigned position and ensure proper disposition of incident documentation as directed by the Documentation Unit.

n. Ensure all equipment is operational prior to each work period.

o. Report any signs/symptoms of extended incident stress, injury, fatigue or illness for yourself or

coworkers to your supervisor.
p. Brief shift replacement on ongoing operations when relieved at operational periods or rotation out.
q. Respond to demobilization orders and brief subordinates regarding demobilization.
r. Prepare personal belongings for demobilization.
s. Return all assigned equipment to appropriate location.
t. Complete Demobilization Check-out process before returning to home base.
u. Participate in After-Action activities as directed.
v. Carry out all assignments as directed.
w. Upon demobilization, notify RESL at incident site and home unit of your safe return.

UNIT LEADER RESPONSIBILITIES

In NIMS ICS, a number of the Unit Leader's responsibilities are common to all functions within the ICS organization. Common responsibilities of Unit Leaders are listed below. These will not be repeated in Unit Leader Position Checklists in subsequent chapters.
a. Review Common Responsibilities in Chapter 2.
b. Upon check-in, receive briefing from Incident Commander, Section Chief, Unit Leader or Branch Director as appropriate.
c. Participate in incident meetings and briefings, as required.
d. Determine current status of unit activities.
e. Determine resource needs.
f. Order additional unit staff, as appropriate.
g. Confirm dispatch and estimated time of arrival of staff and supplies.
h. Assign specific duties to staff and supervise staff.
i. Develop and implement accountability, safety and security measures for personnel and resources.

j. Supervise demobilization of unit, including storage of supplies.

k. Provide Supply Unit Leader with a list of supplies to be replenished.

l. Maintain unit records, including Unit Log (ICS 214-CG).

m. Individual responders may want to maintain personal log of actions, decisions and events.

n. Carry out all assignments as directed.

CHAPTER 3

OPERATIONAL PLANNING CYCLE, MEETINGS, BRIEFINGS, AND THE ACTION PLANNING PROCESS

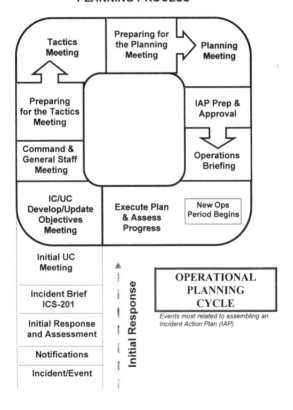

INITIAL RESPONSE AND ASSESSMENT - The period of Initial Response and Assessment occurs in all incidents. Short-term responses, which are small in scope and/or duration (e.g., a few resources working one operational period), can often be coordinated using only ICS-201-CG (Incident Briefing Form).

INCIDENT BRIEFING (ICS-201) - During the transfer-of-command process, an ICS-201-formatted briefing provides the incoming Incident Commander (IC)/Unified Command (UC) with basic information regarding the incident situation and the resources allotted to the incident. Most importantly it functions as the Incident Action Plan (IAP) for the initial response and remains in force and continues to develop (updated) until the response ends or the Planning Section generates the incident's first IAP. It is also suitable for briefing individuals newly assigned to the Command and General Staff, incoming tactical resources, as well as needed assessment briefings for the staff.

ICS-201-CG facilitates documentation of the current situation, initial response objectives, current and planned actions, resources assigned and requested, on-scene organization structure and incident potential. This form is essential for future planning and the effective management of initial response activities.

When:	New IC/UC; staff briefing as required
Facilitator:	Current IC/UC or (PSC if available)
Attendees:	Prospective IC/UC; Command and General Staff, as available

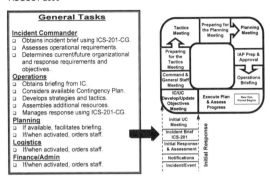

General Tasks

Incident Commander
- Obtains incident brief using ICS-201-CG.
- Assesses operational requirements.
- Determines current/future organizational and response requirements and objectives.

Operations
- Obtains briefing from IC.
- Considers available Contingency Plan.
- Develops strategies and tactics.
- Assembles additional resources.
- Manages response using ICS-201-CG.

Planning
- If available, facilitates briefing.
- If/when activated, orders staff.

Logistics
- If/when activated, orders staff.

Finance/Admin
- If/when activated, orders staff.

Incident Briefing (ICS-201) Agenda:

Using ICS-201-CG as an outline, include:

1. Current situation (note territory, exposures, safety concerns, etc.; use map/charts).
2. Initial objectives and priorities.
3. Current and planned actions.
4. Current on-scene organization.
5. Resource assignments.
6. Resources en-route and/or ordered.
7. Facilities established.
8. Incident potential.

INITIAL UNIFIED COMMAND MEETING - Provides UC officials with an opportunity to discuss and concur on important issues prior to the Unified Command Objectives Meeting. The meeting should be brief and all important decisions and direction documented. Prior to the meeting, IC's should have an opportunity to review and prepare to address the agenda items. The results of this meeting will help to guide the overall response efforts.

When: The UC is formed prior to the first meeting.
Facilitator: UC member or PSC (if available).
Attendees: Only ICs that will comprise the UC, DOCL.

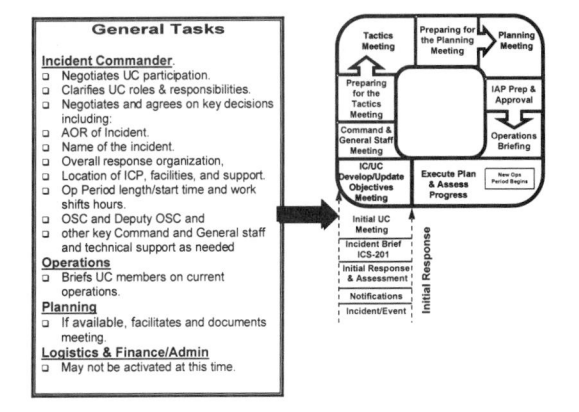

Initial Unified Command Meeting Agenda:
1. Meeting brought to order, cover ground rules and reviews agenda.
2. Validate makeup of newly formed UC, based on Chapter 5 criteria.
3. Clarify UC Roles and Responsibilities.
4. Review agency policies.
5. Negotiate and agree on Key Decisions which may

include:
   a. UC jurisdictional boundaries and focus (Area of Responsibility (AOR)).
   b. Name of incident.
   c. Overall response organization, including integration of assisting and cooperating agencies.
   d. Location of Incident Command Post (if not already identified) and other critical facilities, as appropriate.
   e. Operational period length/start time and work shift hours.
   f. Best-qualified Operations Section Chief and Deputy.
   g. Other key Command and General staff assignments and technical support as needed.
6. Summarize and document key decisions.

UNIFIED COMMAND OBJECTIVES MEETING (Sometimes called STRATEGY MEETING) - The UC will set response priorities, identify any limitations and constraints, develop incident objectives and establish guidelines for the IMT to follow. For reoccurring meetings, all products will be reviewed and updated as needed. Products resulting from this meeting along with decisions and direction from the Initial UC meeting will be presented at the Command and General Staff Meeting.

When:	Prior to Command and General Staff Meeting.
Facilitator:	IC/UC Member or PSC (if available).
Attendees:	IC/UC Members; Selected Command and General Staff as appropriate, DOCL.

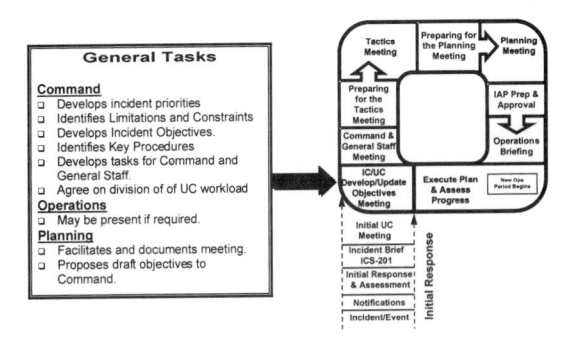

General Tasks

Command
- Develops incident priorities
- Identifies Limitations and Constraints
- Develops Incident Objectives.
- Identifies Key Procedures
- Develops tasks for Command and General Staff.
- Agree on division of of UC workload

Operations
- May be present if required.

Planning
- Facilitates and documents meeting.
- Proposes draft objectives to Command.

Unified Command Objectives Meeting Agenda:

1. PSC brings meeting to order, conducts roll call, covers ground rules and reviews agenda.
2. Review and/or update key decisions.
3. Develop or review/update response Priorities, Limitations and Constraints.
4. Develop or review Incident Objectives.
5. Develop or review/update Key Procedures which may include:
   a. Managing sensitive information,
   b. Information flow
   c. Resource ordering,
   d. Cost sharing and cost accounting, and
   e. Operational security issues.
6. Develop or review/update tasks for Command and General Staff to accomplish (ICS-233-CG).
7. Review, document and/or resolve status of any open actions (ICS-233-CG).
8. Agree on division of UC workload.
9. Prepare for the Command and General Staff Meeting.

COMMAND AND GENERAL STAFF MEETING –

At the Command and General Staff Meeting, IC/UC will present their decisions and management direction to the Command and General Staff Members. This meeting should clarify and help to ensure understanding among the core IMT members on the decisions, objectives, priorities, procedures and functional assignments (tasks) that the UC has discussed and reached agreement on. Ensuing Command and General Staff Meetings will cover any changes in Command direction, review Open Actions and status of assigned tasks (ICS-233-CG).

When:	Prior to Tactics Meeting.
Facilitator:	PSC.
Attendees:	IC/UC Members, Command and General Staff, SITL, and DOCL

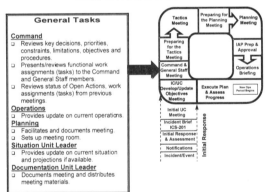

General Tasks

Command
- Reviews key decisions, priorities, constraints, limitations, objectives and procedures.
- Presents/reviews functional work assignments (tasks) to the Command and General Staff members.
- Reviews status of Open Actions, work assignments (tasks) from previous meetings.

Operations
- Provides update on current operations.

Planning
- Facilitates and documents meeting.
- Sets up meeting room.

Situation Unit Leader
- Provides update on current situation and projections if available.

Documentation Unit Leader
- Documents meeting and distributes meeting materials.

Command and General Staff Meeting Agenda:
1. PSC brings meeting to order, conducts roll call, covers ground rules and reviews agenda.
2. SITL conducts situation status briefing.
3. IC/UC
    a. Provides comments.

    b. Reviews key decisions, priorities, constraints and limitations (if new or changed).

    c. Discusses incident objectives,

    d. Reviews key procedures (if new or changed), and

    e. Assigns or reviews functional tasks/open actions (ICS-233-CG).

4. PSC facilitates open discussion to clarify priorities, objectives, assignments, issues, concerns and open actions/tasks.

5. IC/UC provides closing comments.

PREPARING FOR THE TACTICS MEETING – During this phase of the Operational Planning Cycle, the OSC/PSC begin the work of preparing for the upcoming Tactics Meeting. They review incident objectives to determine those that are OSC responsibility and consider Command priorities. They may draft a Work Analysis Matrix (ICS-334-CG) which helps document strategies and tactics to meet those objectives assigned, and should draft an Operational Planning Worksheet (ICS-215-CG) and an Operations Section organization chart for the next operational period. Also, the SOFR should begin to develop the Hazard Risk Analysis Worksheet (ICS-215a-CG). The PSC should facilitate/support this process to the greatest extent possible to ensure that the material, information, resources, etc. to be presented in the Tactics Meeting is organized and accurate.

When:	Prior to Tactics Meeting.
Facilitator:	PSC facilitates process.
Attendees:	None. This is not a meeting but a period of time.

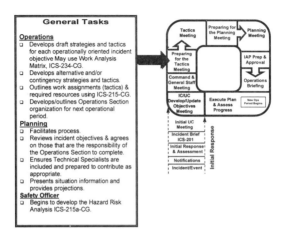

General Tasks

Operations
- Develops draft strategies and tactics for each operationally oriented incident objective May use Work Analysis Matrix, ICS-234-CG.
- Develops alternative and/or contingency strategies and tactics.
- Outlines work assignments (tactics) & required resources using ICS-215-CG.
- Develops/outlines Operations Section organization for next operational period.

Planning
- Facilitates process.
- Reviews incident objectives & agrees on those that are the responsibility of the Operations Section to complete.
- Ensures Technical Specialists are included and prepared to contribute as appropriate.
- Presents situation information and provides projections.

Safety Officer
- Begins to develop the Hazard Risk Analysis ICS-215a-CG.

TACTICS MEETING - This 30-minute meeting produces operational input needed to support the IAP. The OSC may present the Work Analysis Matrix (ICS-234-CG), if completed and will present the draft Operational Planning Worksheet (ICS-215-CG). The proposed Operations Section organization will also be presented by OSC and solidified. The SOFR will present the draft Hazard Risk Analysis Worksheet (ICS-215a-CG). OSC/PSC will solicit input of attendees in order to refine these draft products for full staff approval at the Planning Meeting.

When: Prior to Planning Meeting.
Facilitator: PSC.
Attendees: PSC, OSC, LSC, RESL, SITL, SOFR, DOCL, COML, THSP (as needed).

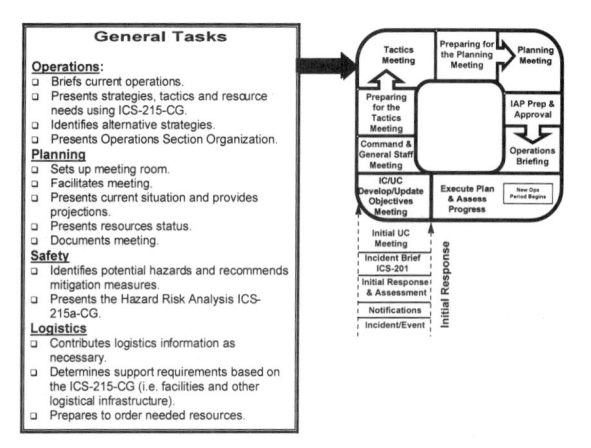

General Tasks

Operations:
- Briefs current operations.
- Presents strategies, tactics and resource needs using ICS-215-CG.
- Identifies alternative strategies.
- Presents Operations Section Organization.

Planning
- Sets up meeting room.
- Facilitates meeting.
- Presents current situation and provides projections.
- Presents resources status.
- Documents meeting.

Safety
- Identifies potential hazards and recommends mitigation measures.
- Presents the Hazard Risk Analysis ICS-215a-CG.

Logistics
- Contributes logistics information as necessary.
- Determines support requirements based on the ICS-215-CG (i.e. facilities and other logistical infrastructure).
- Prepares to order needed resources.

Tactics Meeting Agenda:

1. PSC brings meeting to order, conducts roll call, covers ground rules and reviews agenda.
2. SITL reviews the current & projected incident situation.
3. PSC reviews incident operational objectives and ensures accountability for each.
4. OSC reviews, if completed, the Work Analysis Matrix (ICS-234-CG) strategy and tactics.
5. OSC reviews and/or completes the Operational Planning Worksheet (ICS-215-CG) which addresses work assignments, resource commitments, contingencies and needed support facilities, i.e., Staging Areas.
6. OSC reviews and/or completes Operations Section organization chart.
7. SOFR reviews and/or completes the Hazard Risk Analysis Worksheet (ICS-215a-CG) and identifies and resolves any critical safety issues.

8. LSC discusses and resolves any logistics issues.
9. PSC validates connectivity of tactics and operational objectives.

PREPARING FOR THE PLANNING MEETING

The Command and General Staffs prepare for the upcoming Planning Meeting. The PSC ensures the material, information, resources, etc., used or discussed in the Planning Meeting are prepared and ready for presentation during the meeting.

When: Prior to the Planning Meeting.
Facilitator: PSC facilitates process.
Attendees: None. This is <u>not</u> a meeting but a period of time.

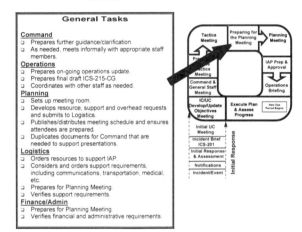

General Tasks

Command
- Prepares further guidance/clarification.
- As needed, meets informally with appropriate staff members.

Operations
- Prepares on-going operations update.
- Prepares final draft ICS-215-CG.
- Coordinates with other staff as needed.

Planning
- Sets up meeting room.
- Develops resource, support and overhead requests and submits to Logistics.
- Publishes/distributes meeting schedule and ensures attendees are prepared.
- Duplicates documents for Command that are needed to support presentations.

Logistics
- Orders resources to support IAP.
- Considers and orders support requirements, including communications, transportation, medical, etc.
- Prepares for Planning Meeting.
- Verifies support requirements.

Finance/Admin
- Prepares for Planning Meeting.
- Verifies financial and administrative requirements.

PLANNING MEETING - This meeting provides an overview of the tactical plan to achieve Command's current direction, priorities and objectives. The OSC will present the proposed plan to the Command and General Staff for review and comment. OSC will discuss strategy and tactics that were considered and chosen to best meet command's direction for the next operational period. The OSC will also briefly discuss how the incident will be managed along with work assignments and resources and support required to implement the proposed plan. This meeting provides the opportunity for Command and General Staff to discuss and resolve any issues and concerns prior to assembling the IAP. After review and updates are made, planning meeting attendees commit to support the plan.

When:	After the Tactics Meeting.
Facilitator:	PSC.
Attendees:	IC/UC, Command Staff, General Staff, SITL, DOCL and THSP (as required).

General Tasks

Command
- Ensures all of Command's direction, priorities and objectives have been met.
- Provides further direction and resolves differences as needed.
- Gives tacit approval of proposed plan.

Operations
- Provides overview of current OPS.
- Presents plan of action including; strategies, tactics, contingencies, resources, organization structure and overall management considerations i.e. divisions/groups etc.

Planning
- Facilitates meeting.
- Briefs current situation.
- Provides projections.
- Documents meeting.

Logistics
- Briefs logistical support/services and resource ordering status.
- Discusses operational facility issues.

Finance/Admin
- Briefs administrative and financial status/projections, etc.

Command Staff
- Discusses and resolves any Safety, Liaison and Media considerations and issues.

Planning Meeting Agenda:

1. PSC brings meeting to order, conducts roll call, covers ground rules and reviews agenda.
2. IC/UC provides opening remarks.
3. SITL provides briefing on current situation, resources at risk, weather/sea forecast and incident projections.
4. PSC reviews Command's incident priorities, decisions and objectives.
5. OSC provides briefing on current operations followed with an overview on the proposed plan including strategy, tactics/work assignments (ICS-215-CG), resource commitment, contingencies, Operations Section organization structure and needed support facilities, i.e., Staging Areas.
6. PSC reviews proposed plan to ensure that Command's priorities and operational objectives are met.
7. PSC reviews and validates responsibility for any open actions/tasks (ICS-233-CG) and management objectives.
8. PSC conducts round robin of Command and General Staff members to solicit their final input and commitment to the proposed plan:
   a. LSC covers transport, communications and supply updates and issues,
   b. FSC covers fiscal issues.
   c. SOFR covers safety issues,
   d. PIO covers public affairs and public information issues,
   e. LNO covers interagency issues and
   f. INTO covers intelligence issues.
9. PSC requests Command's tacit approval of the plan as presented. IC/UC may provide final comments.
10. PSC issues assignments to appropriate IMT members for developing IAP support documentation along with deadlines.

INCIDENT ACTION PLAN PREPARATION AND APPROVAL –

Appropriate IMT members must immediately complete the assigned task/products that are needed to include in the IAP. These products must meet the deadline as set by the PSC so that planning can assemble the IAP components. The deadline must be early enough to permit timely IC/UC review, approval, and duplication of sufficient copies for the Operations Briefing and other IMT members.

When: Immediately following the Planning Meeting, the PSC assigns the deadline for products.

Facilitator: PSC facilitates process.

Attendees: None. This is <u>not</u> a meeting but a period of time.

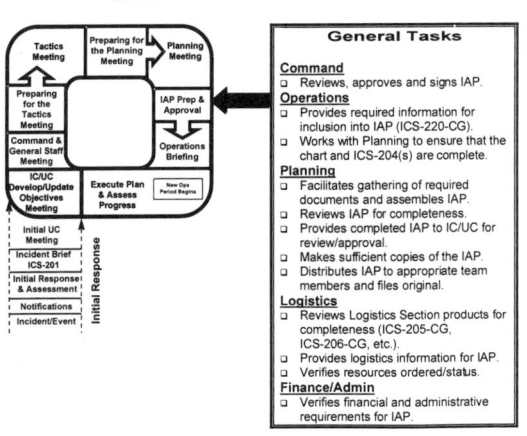

General Tasks

Command
- Reviews, approves and signs IAP.

Operations
- Provides required information for inclusion into IAP (ICS-220-CG).
- Works with Planning to ensure that the chart and ICS-204(s) are complete.

Planning
- Facilitates gathering of required documents and assembles IAP.
- Reviews IAP for completeness.
- Provides completed IAP to IC/UC for review/approval.
- Makes sufficient copies of the IAP.
- Distributes IAP to appropriate team members and files original.

Logistics
- Reviews Logistics Section products for completeness (ICS-205-CG, ICS-206-CG, etc.).
- Provides logistics information for IAP.
- Verifies resources ordered/status.

Finance/Admin
- Verifies financial and administrative requirements for IAP.

IAP Common Components   Primary Responsibility

1.	Incident Objectives (ICS-202-CG).	RESL
2.	Organization List/Chart (ICS-203/207-CG).	RESL
3.	Assignment List (ICS-204-CG).	RESL
4.	Communication Plan (ICS-205-CG).	COML
5.	Medical Plan (ICS-206-CG).	MEDL
6.	Site Safety Plan (ICS-208-CG).	SOFR
7.	Incident Map/Chart.	SITL
8.	Weather, tide forecast	SITL

Optional Components (use as pertinent):

1.	Air Operations Summary (ICS-220-CG)	AOBD
2.	Demobilization Plan	DMOB
3.	Transportation Plan	GSUL
4.	Decontamination Plan	THSP
5.	Waste Management or Disposal Plan	THSP
6.	Other Plans and/or documents, as required	

OPERATIONS BRIEFING - This 30-minute, or less, briefing presents the IAP to the Operations Section oncoming shift supervisors. After this briefing has occurred and during shift change, off-going supervisors should be interviewed by their relief and by OSC in order to validate IAP effectiveness. The Division/Group Supervisor may make last minute adjustments to tactics over which they have purview. Similarly, a supervisor may reallocate resources within that Division/Group to adapt to changing conditions.

When: Approximately one hour prior to shift change.
Facilitator: PSC.
Attendees: IC/UC, Command and General Staff, Branch Directors, Division/Group Supervisors, Task Force/Strike Team Leaders (if possible), Unit Leaders, others as appropriate.

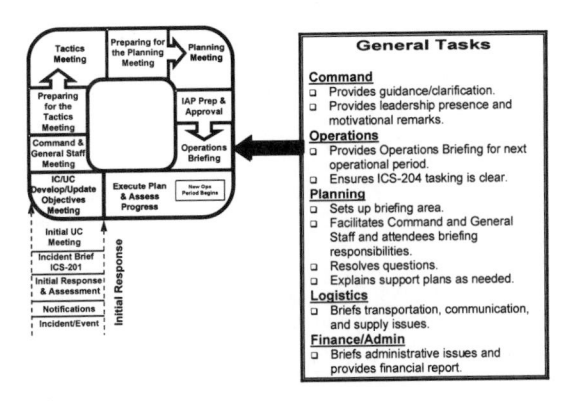

Operations Briefing Agenda:

1. PSC opens briefing, covers ground rules, agenda and takes roll call of Command and General Staff and Operations personnel required to attend.

2. PSC reviews IC/UC objectives and changes to the IAP, i.e., pen and ink changes.

3. IC/UC provides remarks.

4. SITL conducts Situation Briefing.

5. OSC discusses current response actions and accomplishments.

6. OSC briefs Operations Section personnel.

7. LSC covers transport, communications and supply updates.

8. FSC covers fiscal issues.

9. SOFR covers safety issues, PIO covers public affairs and public information issues, LNO covers interagency issues and INTO covers intelligence issues.

10. PSC solicits final comments and adjourns briefing.

ASSESS PROGRESS – Assessment is an on-going continuous process to help adjust current operations and help plan for future operations. Following the briefing, and shift change, all Command and General Staff Section Chiefs will review the incident response progress and make recommendations to the IC/UC in preparation for the next IC/UC Objectives Meeting. This feedback/information is continuously gathered from various sources, including Field Observers, responder debriefs, stakeholders, etc. IC/UC should encourage Command and General Staff to get out of the ICP and view first hand the areas of the incident they are supporting.

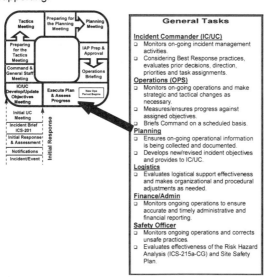

General Tasks

Incident Commander (IC/UC)
- Monitors on-going incident management activities.
- Considering Best Response practices, evaluates prior decisions, direction, priorities and task assignments.

Operations (OPS)
- Monitors on-going operations and make strategic and tactical changes as necessary.
- Measures/ensures progress against assigned objectives.
- Briefs Command on a scheduled basis.

Planning
- Ensures on-going operational information is being collected and documented.
- Develops new/revised incident objectives and provides to IC/UC.

Logistics
- Evaluates logistical support effectiveness and makes organizational and procedural adjustments as needed.

Finance/Admin
- Monitors ongoing operations to ensure accurate and timely administrative and financial reporting.

Safety Officer
- Monitors ongoing operations and corrects unsafe practices.
- Evaluates effectiveness of the Risk Hazard Analysis (ICS-215a-CG) and Site Safety Plan.

SPECIAL PURPOSE MEETINGS

Special Purpose meetings are most applicable to larger incidents requiring an **Operational Period Planning Cycle**, but may also be useful during the **Initial Response Phase**.

BUSINESS MANAGEMENT MEETING – The purpose of this meeting is to develop and update the Business Management Plan for finance and logistical support. The agenda could include: documentation issues, cost sharing, cost analysis, finance requirements, resource procurement, and financial summary data. Attendees normally include: FSC, COST, PROC, LSC, SITL, and DOCL.

AGENCY REPRESENTATIVE MEETING - This meeting is held to update Agency Representatives and ensure that they can support the IAP. It is conducted by the LNO, and attended by Agency Representatives. It is most appropriately held shortly after the Planning Meeting in order to present the plan (IAP) for the next operational period. It allows for minor changes should the plan not meet the expectations of the Agency Representatives.

MEDIA BRIEFING - This meeting is normally conducted at the Joint Information Center (JIC). Its purpose is to brief the media and the public on the most current and accurate facts. It is set up by the PIO, moderated by a UC spokesperson, and features selected spokespersons. Spokespersons should be prepared by the PIO to address anticipated issues. The briefing should be well-planned, organized, and scheduled to meet media's needs.

TECHNICAL SPECIALIST MEETING – Meetings to gather THSP input to IAP.

DEMOBILIZATION PLANNING MEETING – This meeting is held to gather functional requirements from Command, Command Staff and General Staff that would be included in the incident Demobilization Plan. Functional requirements would include: safety, logistic, and fiscal considerations and release priorities that would be addressed in the plan. Attendees normally include: Command, OSC, PSC, LSC, FSC, LNO, SOFR, INTO PIO and DMOB. The DMOB then prepares a draft Demobilization Plan to include the functional requirements and distributes to Command, Command Staff and General Staff for review and comment.

THIS PAGE INTENTIONALLY LEFT BLANK

CHAPTER 4

KEY DECISIONS, PRIORITIES, RESPONSE OBJECTIVES AND STAFF ASSIGNMENTS

References:
- (a) Incident Commander Job Aid
- (b) Area Command Job Aid

INTRODUCTION

Incident Commander(s) are responsible for providing direction and guidance to the Incident Management Team (IMT). Command must analyze the overall requirements of the incident and determine the most appropriate direction for the management team to follow during the response. This is accomplished by making key decisions, setting priorities, developing response objectives and assigning work (tasks) to primary staff within the IMT. This chapter can be used by Command to help facilitate their responsibilities. The information/examples provided can be used as is or modified in response to specific risk applications. See Reference (a) for more information on key Command decisions, priorities, response objectives and staff assignments.

Example Decisions:
o   Incident name.
o   Organizations/agencies that will be represented in Unified Command.
o   Integration of other supporting and cooperating organizations/agencies.
o   Support facilities and locations (ICP, Base, JIC etc.).
o   Operational period and hours of operation.
o   Issuing delegation of authority to staff.
o   Critical information reporting process.
o   Managing sensitive information.
o   Resource ordering, cost sharing and cost accounting.
o   Operational security issues.
o   Staffing of primary positions (OSC and Deputy).
o   Incident Response Priorities.
o   IMT Procedures/function.
o   How Command will function.

Example Incident Priorities:
o   Safety of responders and the public.
o   Threat to Homeland Security.
o   Minimize adverse impact on the environment.
o   Restoration of the transportation infrastructure/ maritime commerce.
o   Minimize further loss of property.
o   Investigation and apprehension of those responsible.
o   Reduce/prevent further threat/attack.

Example Incident Objectives

<u>Safety</u>:
o   Provide for the safety and welfare of citizens and response personnel.
o   Provide for the safety and security of responders as well as maximize the protection of public health and welfare.
o   Identify safety and risk management factors and monitor for compliance for both the public and responders.
o   Implement practices that allow for the safety and welfare of the passengers and non-essential crew.
o   Conduct Operational Risk Assessment and ensure controls are in place to protect responders and the public.

<u>Search and Rescue</u>:
o   Locate and evacuate all passengers and crew.
o   Evacuate victims to medical transfer areas or facilities once rescued from immediate peril.
o   Establish medical triage along with transport to hospital.
o   Complete triage of injured passengers and crew and transport to hospital.
o   Conduct joint agency SAR efforts.
o   Conduct Urban Search and Rescue.
o   Account for and provide temporary shelter for displaced passengers and crew.
o   Complete accountability for all passengers and crew.

<u>Fire/Salvage</u>:
o   Commence fire fighting operations and contain, extinguish and overhaul fire.
o   Conduct damage/stability assessment; develop and implement a salvage plan.
o   Implement the salvage and tow plan.

Port, Waterways, and Coastal Security/Law Enforcement:

o   Implement security awareness measures including evaluation of changes in incident effects, response conditions, and secondary threats, including potential targeting of first responders and contamination.

o   Implement measures to isolate, contain and stabilize the incident, including establishment and adjustment of security perimeters.

o   Implement agency and maritime community security plans, including Area Maritime Security Plans (AMSP), to deter and prevent multiple security incidents.

o   Establish incident security plan including identification badges and other scene control measures.

o   Implement scene integrity and evidence preservation procedures.

o   Implement procedures that ensure a coordinated effort is in place for investigation, evidence collection, storage and disposal.

o   Investigate cause of incident.

o   Identify and implement witness/passenger recovery location(s).

o   Establish incident security plan including access documentation (e.g. badge control procedures) and other access control measures.

o   Establish and continue enforcement of safety/ security zones.

o   Establish/conduct shoreline security to coincide with incident activities and enhanced prevention requirements.

o   Perform maritime law enforcement as required.

o   Request FAA Implement air space closure and monitoring for compliance.

4-4

KEY DECISIONS/OBJECTIVES   KEY DECISIONS/OBJECTIVES

Waterways Management:
o   Conduct port assessment and establish priorities for facilitating commerce.
o   Develop/implement transit plan to include final destination/berth for vessel(s).
o   Identify safe refuge/berth for impacted vessels.
o   Establish and maintain close coordination for possible movement of Homeland or National Security assets (Navy).

Oil/HAZMAT Spills:
o   Initiate actions to control the source and minimize the volume released.
o   Determine oil/hazmat fate and effect (trajectories) identify sensitive areas, develop strategies for protection and conduct pre-impact shoreline debris removal.
o   Contain and recover spilled material (Oil/Hazmat).
o   Conduct an assessment and initiate shoreline cleanup efforts.
o   Remove product from impacted areas.
o   Conduct efforts to effectively contain, clean up, recover and dispose of spilled product.

Environmental:
o   Provide protection of environmental sensitive areas including wildlife and historic properties.
o   Identify and maximize the protection of environmental sensitive areas.
o   Identify threatened species and prepare to recover and rehabilitate injured wildlife.
o   Investigate the potential for and if feasible, utilize alternative technologies to support response efforts.

<u>Management</u>:
o   Manage a coordinated interagency response effort that reflects the makeup of Unified Command.
o   Establish an appropriate IMT organization that can effectively meet the initial and long term challenges required to mitigate the incident.
o   Identify all appropriate agency/organization mandates, practices, and protocols for inclusion in the overall response effort.
o   Identify and minimize social, political and economic adverse effects.
o   Implement a coordinated response with law enforcement and other responding agencies including EOC(s) and the JFO.
o   Evaluate all planned actions to determine potential impacts on social, political and economic entities.
o   Identify competing response activities (LE and Mitigation) to ensure that they are closely coordinated.
o   Identify and establish incident support facilities to support interagency response efforts.
o   Keep the public, stakeholders and the media informed of response activities.
o   Ensure appropriate financial accounting practices are established and adhered to.
o   Establish internal/external resource ordering procedures are established and adhered to.
o   Establish an incident documentation system.
o   Establish an appropriate structure to facilitate communications with stakeholders and agency/organization coordination facilities.

Example Tasks/Work Assignments:
Incident Management Team members expect Command to assign them specific tasks based on the unique characteristics of an incident. Common tasks

that are normally performed by the staff during responses should not be addressed as tasks. The Operations Section Chief normally receives tasks (work assignments) from Command in the form of incident objectives. Some examples of common tasks (work assignments):

Safety Officer:
o   Develop a site safety plan, including support facilities and monitor for compliance.
o   Report any serious incidents, accidents, or injuries immediately to command.
o   Work closely with Logistics to ensure that appropriate communications are in place to support the response effort.

Public Information Officer:
o   Develop a media strategy, Review strategy with Command prior to implementation.
o   Establish contact with other Public Information personnel.
o   Locate and establish a JIC.
o   Provide talking points to Command for press briefings, VIP visits and town hall meetings.
o   Keep Command informed of any potential adverse political, social, and economic impacts.

Liaison Officer:
o   Develop an action plan to ensure communication and coordination with appropriate stakeholders and submit draft of plan to Command for review and approval.
o   Keep Command informed of any stakeholder adverse feelings/relationships that may develop.

Intelligence Officer:
o   Identify critical intelligence needs and develop intelligence flow plan and brief IMT.

o Ensure that all requests for information (RFI's) are sent and the Command is briefed on all Field Intelligence Reports (FIR).
o Be central point of coordination for all interagency intelligence organizations: Field Intelligence Support Teams, Joint Terrorism Task Forces, Intelligence Fusion Centers, etc.
o Screen intelligence information for OPSEC/Security Sensitive Information (SSI) classification.

Planning:
o Ensure that all off-site information reporting is approved by Command prior to release.
o Develop a contingency plan for sustaining long-term IMT staffing.
o Brief IMT staff on document control system, including handling and storing secure documents.
o Provide all documents that need review or approval by Command at least one hour prior to implementation or release.

Finance/Admin:
o Provide Command with a summary daily cost estimate.
o Establish a claims system and brief the IMT on the process.
o Advise Command of unusual high cost specialized equipment use.

Logistics:
o Develop and brief the IMT on the internal/external resource ordering process and monitor for compliance.
o Ensure that appropriate security is established at each incident support facility.
o Develop a plan; establish secure communication for both internal and external use and brief IMT staff.

CHAPTER 5

UNIFIED COMMAND

Reference:
  (a) Incident Commander Job Aid

INTRODUCTION

Unified Command (UC) is an expansion of the ICS organization. To be a member of the UC you must have authority and jurisdiction. UC members may also include agencies, organizations or private industries bringing large amounts of tactical and support resources to the table. The need for UC is brought about when an incident impacts the jurisdictional or functional responsibility of more than one agency. As a component of ICS, the UC is a structure that brings together the "Incident Commanders" of all major organizations that have jurisdictional responsibility for the incident to coordinate an effective response while carrying out their own agencies jurisdictional responsibilities. UC links the responding organizations to the incident and provides a forum for these agencies to make consensus decisions. Under UC, the various jurisdictions and/or agencies and non-government responders may blend together throughout the organization to create an integrated response team.

The need for UC arises when incidents:
- Cross geographic boundaries (e.g., two states, international boundaries);
- Involve various governmental levels (e.g., Federal, state, local,);
- Impact functional responsibilities (e.g., Search and Rescue, fire, oil spill, EMS); or
- Some combination of the above.

UC Make Up:

Actual UC makeup for a specific incident will be determined on a case-by-case basis taking into account:

(1) The specifics of the incident;
(2) Determinations outlined in existing response plans; or
(3) Decisions reached during the initial meeting of the UC. The makeup of the UC may change as an incident progresses in order to account for changes in the situation.

UC is a team effort, but to be effective the number of personnel should be kept as small as possible. A well-defined process requires the UC to set clear objectives to guide the on-scene response resources.

UC is responsible for overall management of the incident. UC directs incident activities, including development and implementation of overall objectives and strategies, and approves ordering and releasing of resources. UC is not a "decision by committee". The principals are there to command the response to an incident. Time is of the essence. UC should develop synergy based on the significant capabilities that are brought by the various representatives. There should be personal acknowledgement of each representative's unique capabilities, a shared understanding of the situation, and agreement on the common objectives. With the different perspectives on UC comes the risk of disagreements, most of which can be resolved through the understanding of the underlying issues. Contentious issues may arise, but the UC framework provides a forum and a process to resolve problems and find solutions.

5-2

A cooperative attitude and a thorough understanding are essential. as is a thorough understanding of the ICS Operating Cycle. Nevertheless, situations may arise where consensus agreement may not be reachable. In such instances, the UC member representing the agency with the most jurisdictional responsibility would normally be deferred to for the final decision.

The bottom line is that UC has certain responsibilities as noted above. Failure to provide clear incident objectives and response direction means that UC has failed. While the UC structure is an excellent vehicle (and the only nationally recognized vehicle) for coordination, cooperation, and communication, the duly authorized representatives must make the system work successfully. A strong Command – a single IC or UC – is essential to an effective response.

In order to keep the UC small in numbers; and therefore efficient, it is recommended that one agency in the State or Federal government should be the lead agency to coordinate activities and actions within the State/Federal agencies involved. Specific representatives of various agencies should be encouraged to participate on the response team in the functions that best suit their expertise.

The UC may assign Deputy Incident Commander(s) to assist in carrying out IC and/or UC responsibilities. UC members may also be assigned individual legal and administrative support from their own organizations.

To be considered for inclusion as a UC representative, the involved organization:

1. Must have jurisdictional authority or functional responsibility under a law or ordinance for the incident; and,
2. Must have incident or response operations impact on your organization's Area Of Responsibility (AOR); and,
3. Must be specifically charged by law or ordinance with commanding, coordinating or managing a major aspect of the incident response; and,
4. Should have the resources to support participation in the response organization.

UC representatives must be able to:

- Agree on incident objectives and priorities;
- Have the capability to sustain a 24-hour-7-day-a-week commitment to the incident;
- Have the authority to commit agency or company resources to the incident;
- Have the authority to spend agency or company funds;
- Agree on constraints/limitations, priorities, decisions and procedures;
- Agree on an incident response organization;
- Agree on the appropriate Command and General Staff position assignments to ensure clear direction for on-scene tactical resources;
- Commit to speak with "one voice" through the PIO or JIC, if established;
- Agree on managing sensitive information and operational security issues;
- Agree on logistical support including resource ordering procedures; and
- Agree on cost-sharing and cost accounting procedures, as appropriate.

5-4

It is important to note that participation in UC occurs <u>without</u> any agency abdicating authority, responsibility, or accountability.

What if your agency is not represented in UC but is involved in the response effort?
Here is how to ensure your organization's concerns or issues are addressed:

- Serve as an agency or company representative who has direct contact with the Liaison Officer (LNO).
- Provide stakeholder input to the LNO (for environmental, economic, social, or political issues).
- Serve as a Technical Specialist in the Planning Section.
- Provide input directly to a member of UC.

THIS PAGE INTENTIONALLY LEFT BLANK

CHAPTER 6

COMMAND STAFF

ORGANIZATION CHART

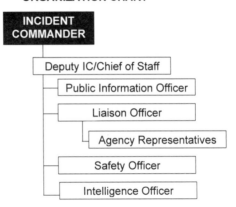

References:
- (a) Incident Commander Job Aid
- (b) Public Information Officer Job Aid
- (c) Joint Information Center Job Aid
- (d) Liaison Officer Job Aid
- (e) Safety Officer Job Aid
- (f) Intelligence Officer Job Aid

POSITION CHECKLISTS

INCIDENT COMMANDER (IC) – The IC's responsibility is the overall management of the incident. On many incidents, the command activity is carried out by a single IC. The IC is selected based on qualifications and experience. The IC Job Aid (reference (a)) should be reviewed regarding the responsibilities and duties of the IC.

The IC may have Deputy IC's, who may be from the same agency or from an assisting agency. The Deputy IC must have the same qualifications as the person for whom they work, as they must be ready to take over that position at any time. When span of control becomes an issue for the IC, a Deputy IC/Chief of Staff may be assigned to manage the Command Staff.

The major responsibilities of the IC are:
   a. Review Common Responsibilities in Chapter 2.
   b. Obtain a briefing from the prior IC (201 Briefing).
   c. Determine Incident Objectives and general direction for managing the incident.
   d. Establish priorities.
   e. Establish an ICP.
   f. Brief Command Staff and Section Chiefs.
   g. Establish an appropriate organization.
   h. Ensure planning meetings are scheduled as required.
   i. Approve and authorize the implementation of an IAP.
   j. Ensure that adequate safety measures are in place.
   k. Coordinate activity for all Command and General Staff.
   l. Coordinate with key people and officials.
   m. Approve requests for additional resources or for

6-2

COMMAND STAFF   **COMMAND STAFF**

the release of resources.
n. Keep agency administrator informed of incident status.
o. Approve the use of trainees, volunteers, and auxiliary personnel.
p. Authorize release of information to the news media.
q. Ensure Incident Status Summary (ICS 209-CG) is completed and forwarded to appropriate higher authority.
r. Order the demobilization of the incident when appropriate.
s. Maintain Unit Log (ICS 214-CG).

PUBLIC INFORMATION OFFICER (PIO) – The PIO is responsible for developing and releasing information about the incident to the news media, to incident personnel, and to other appropriate agencies and organizations.

Only one primary PIO will be assigned for each incident, including incidents operating under UC and multi-jurisdiction incidents. The PIO may have assistants as necessary, and the assistants may also represent assisting agencies or jurisdictions. The PIO and Joint Information Center (JIC) Job Aids (references (b) and (c)) should be reviewed regarding the organization and duties of the PIO.

Agencies have different policies and procedures relative to the handling of public information. The following are the major responsibilities of the PIO, which would generally apply on any incident.
The major responsibilities of the PIO are:
a. Review Common Responsibilities in Chapter 2.
b. Determine from the IC if there are any limits on information release.

c. Develop material for use in media briefings.
d. Obtain IC approval of media releases.
e. Inform media and conduct media briefings.
f. Arrange for tours and other interviews or briefings that may be required.
g. Manage a Joint Information Center (JIC) if established.
h. Obtain media information that may be useful to incident planning.
i. Maintain current information summaries and/or displays on the incident and provide information on the status of the incident to assigned personnel.
j. Ensure that all required agency forms, reports and documents are completed prior to demobilization.
k. Brief Command on PIO issues and concerns.
l. Have debriefing session with the IC prior to demobilization.
m. Maintain Unit Log (ICS 214-CG).

LIAISON OFFICER (LNO) – Incidents that are multi-jurisdictional, or have several agencies involved, may require the establishment of the LNO position on the Command Staff. Only one primary LNO will be assigned for each incident, including incidents operating under UC and multi-jurisdiction incidents.

The LNO may have assistants as necessary, and the assistants may also represent assisting agencies or jurisdictions. The LNO is assigned to the incident to be the contact for assisting and/or cooperating Agency Representatives. The LNO Job Aid (reference (d)) should be reviewed regarding the organization and duties of the LNO.
The major responsibilities of the LNO are:
a. Review Common Responsibilities in Chapter 2.

6-4

b. Be a contact point for Agency Representatives.

c. Maintain a list of assisting and cooperating agencies and Agency Representatives, including name and contact information. Monitor check-in sheets daily to ensure that all Agency Representatives are identified.

d. Assist in establishing and coordinating interagency contacts.

e. Keep agencies supporting the incident aware of incident status.

f. Monitor incident operations to identify current or potential inter-organizational problems.

g. Participate in planning meetings, providing limitations and capability of assisting agency resources.

h. Coordinate response resource needs for Natural Resource Damage Assessment and Restoration (NRDAR) activities with the OSC during oil and HAZMAT responses.

i. Coordinate response resource needs for incident investigation activities with the OSC.

j. Coordinate activities of visiting dignitaries.

k. Ensure that all required agency forms, reports and documents are completed prior to demobilization.

l. Brief Command on agency issues and concerns.

m. Have debriefing session with the IC prior to demobilization.

n. Maintain Unit Log (ICS 214-CG).

AGENCY REPRESENTATIVE (AREP) – In many multi-jurisdiction incidents, an agency or jurisdiction may send an AREP who is not on direct tactical assignment, but is there to assist in coordination efforts.

An AREP is an individual assigned to an incident from an assisting or cooperating agency who has been

6-5

delegated authority to make decisions on matters affecting that agency's participation at the incident. AREP's report to the LNO or to the IC in the absence of a LNO.

The major responsibilities of the AREPs are:

a. Review Common Responsibilities in Chapter 2.

b. Ensure that all agency resources are properly checked in at the incident.

c. Obtain briefing from the LNO or IC.

d. Inform assisting or cooperating agency personnel on the incident that the AREP position for that agency has been filled.

e. Attend briefings and planning meetings as required.

f. Provide input on the use of agency resources unless resource Technical Specialists (THSP) are assigned from the agency.

g. Cooperate fully with the IC and the General Staff on agency involvement at the incident.

h. Ensure the well-being of agency personnel assigned to the incident.

i. Advise the LNO of any special agency needs or requirements.

j. Report to home agency dispatch or headquarters on a pre-arranged schedule.

k. Ensure that all agency personnel and equipment are properly accounted for and released prior to departure.

l. Ensure that all required agency forms, reports and documents are completed prior to demobilization.

m. Have a debriefing session with the LNO or IC before demobilization.

n. Maintain Unit Log (ICS 214-CG).

SAFETY OFFICER (SOFR) – The SOFR function is to develop and recommend measures for assuring personnel safety and to assess and/or anticipate hazardous and unsafe situations. Only one primary SOFR will be assigned for each incident. The SOFR Job Aid (reference (e)) should be reviewed regarding the organization and duties of the SOFR.

The SOFR may have assistants, as necessary, and the assistants may also represent assisting agencies or jurisdictions. Safety assistants may have specific responsibilities, such as air operations, hazardous materials, etc.

The major responsibilities of the SOFR are:

    a.   Review Common Responsibilities in Chapter 2.

    b.   Participate in tactics and planning meetings, and other meetings and briefings as required.

    c.   Identify hazardous situations associated with the incident.

    d.   Review the IAP for safety implications.

    e.   Provide safety advice in the IAP for assigned responders.

    f.   Exercise emergency authority to stop and prevent unsafe acts.

    g.   Investigate accidents that have occurred within the incident area.

    h.   Assign assistants, as needed.

    i.   Review and approve the Medical Plan (ICS 206-CG).

    j.   Develop the Site Safety Plan and publish Site Safety Plan Summary (ICS 208-CG) as required.

    k.   Develop the Work Safety Analysis Worksheet (ICS-215a-CG) as required.

    l.   Ensure that all required agency forms, reports and documents are completed prior to demobilization.

    m.   Brief Command on safety issues and concerns.

    n.   Have debriefing session with the IC prior to demobilization.

o.   Maintain Unit Log (ICS 214-CG).

INTELLIGENCE OFFICER (INTO) – For the U.S. Coast Guard, the intelligence function has been determined to best fit as the INTO. For more information on the Intelligence function, see Chapter 11. The responsibility of the INTO is to provide Command intelligence information that can have a direct impact on the safety of response personnel and influence the disposition of maritime security assets involved in the response.

The major responsibilities of the INTO are:

a.   Review Common Responsibilities in Chapter 2.
b.   Participate in meetings and briefings as required.
c.   Collect and analyze incoming intelligence information from all sources.
d.   Determine the applicability, significance, and reliability of incoming intelligence information.
e.   As requested, provide intelligence briefings to the IC/UC.
f.   Provide intelligence briefings in support of the ICS Planning Cycle.
g.   Provide Situation Unit with periodic updates of intelligence issues that impact the incident response.
h.   Review the IAP for intelligence implications.
i.   Answer intelligence questions and advise Command and General Staff as appropriate.
j.   Supervise, coordinate, and participate in the collection, analysis, processing, and dissemination of intelligence.
k.   Assist in establishing and maintaining systematic, cross-referenced intelligence records and files.
l.   Establish liaison with all participating law enforcement agencies including the CGIS, FBI/JTTF, State and Local police departments.

6-8

m. Conduct first order analysis on all incoming intelligence and fuse all applicable incoming intelligence with current intelligence holdings in preparation for briefings.

n. Prepare all required intelligence reports and plans.

o. As the incident dictates, determine need to implant Intelligence Technical Specialists in the Planning and Operations Sections.

p. Ensure that all required agency forms, reports and documents are completed prior to demobilization.

q. Have debriefing session with the IC prior to demobilization.

r. Maintain Unit Log (ICS 214-CG).

THIS PAGE INTENTIONALLY LEFT BLANK

CHAPTER 7

OPERATIONS SECTION

ORGANIZATION CHART

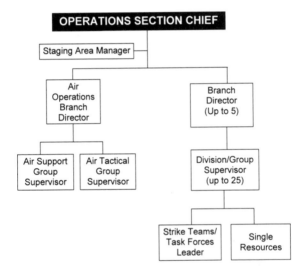

Reference:
(a) Operations Section Chief Job Aid

POSITION CHECKLISTS

OPERATIONS SECTION CHIEF (OSC) – The OSC, a member of the General Staff, is responsible for the management of all tactical operations directly applicable to the primary mission. The OSC will normally be selected from the organization/agency with the most jurisdictional responsibility for the incident.

The OSC activates and supervises organization elements in accordance with the IAP and directs its execution. The OSC also directs the preparation of operational plans; requests or releases resources, monitors operational progress and makes expedient changes to the IAP, as necessary; and reports such to the IC. The OSC Job Aid, Reference (a), should be reviewed regarding the organization and duties of the OSC.

The OSC may have Deputy OSC's, who may be from the same agency or from an assisting agency. The Deputy OSC must have the same qualifications as the person for whom they work, as they must be ready to take over that position at any time. In complex incidents, the OSC may assign a Deputy OSC to supervise on-scene operations (major responsibilities (d) through (k) listed below) while the OSC participates in the incident planning process (major responsibilities (l) through (w) listed below).

The major responsibilities of the OSC are:
  a. Review Common Responsibilities in Chapter 2.
  b. Obtain briefing from IC.
  c. Evaluate and request sufficient Section supervisory staffing for both operational and planning activities.
  d. Supervise Operations Section field personnel.

7-2

e. Implement the IAP for the Operations Section.

f. Evaluate on-scene operations and make adjustments to organization, strategies, tactics, and resources as necessary.

g. Ensure the Resources Unit is advised of changes in the status of resources assigned to the section.

h. Ensure that Operations Section personnel execute work assignments following approved safety practices.

i. Monitor need for and request additional resources to support operations as necessary.

j. Assemble/dissemble task force/strike teams as appropriate.

k. Identify/utilize staging areas.

l. Evaluate and monitor current situation for use in next operational period planning.

m. Convert operational incident objectives into strategic and tactical options. These options may be documented on a Work Analysis Matrix (ICS-234-CG).

n. Coordinate and consult with the PSC, SOFR technical specialists, modeling scenarios, trajectories, etc., on selection of appropriate strategies and tactics to accomplish objectives.

o. Identify kind and number of resources required to support selected strategies.

p. Subdivide work areas into manageable units.

q. Develop work assignments and allocate tactical resources based on strategic requirements (i.e. develop the ICS-215-CG).

r. Coordinate planned activities with the SOFR to ensure compliance with safety practices.

s. Participate in the planning process and the development of the tactical portions (ICS 204-CG and ICS 220-CG) of the IAP.

t. Assist with development of long-range strategic, contingency, and demobilization plans.

7-3

u. Develop recommended list of Section resources to be demobilized and initiate recommendation for release when appropriate.
v. Receive and implement applicable portions of the incident Demobilization Plan.
w. Participate in operational briefings to IMT members as well as briefings to media, and visiting dignitaries.
x. Maintain Unit Log (ICS 214-CG).

BRANCH DIRECTOR (OPBD) – The OPBD's when activated, are under the direction of the OSC and are responsible for the implementation of the portion of the IAP appropriate to the Branches.
The major responsibilities of the OPBD are:

a. Review Common Responsibilities in Chapter 2.
b. Obtain briefing from person relieving.
c. Receive briefing from the OSC.
d. Identify Divisions, Groups, and resources assigned to the Branch.
e. Ensure that Division and/or Group Supervisors (DIVS) have a copy of the IAP.
f. Implement IAP for the Branch.
g. Develop with subordinates alternatives for Branch control operations.
h. Review Division/Group Assignment Lists (ICS 204-CG) for Divisions/Groups within the Branch. Modify lists based on effectiveness of current operations.
i. Assign specific work tasks to DIVS.
j. Supervise Branch operations.
k. Resolve logistic problems reported by subordinates.
l. Attend planning meetings as requested by the OSC.
m. Ensure through chain of command that Resources Unit is advised of changes in the

7-4

status of resources assigned to the Branch.
n. Report to OSC when: the IAP is to be modified; additional resources are needed; surplus resources are available; or hazardous situations or significant events occur.
o. Approve accident and medical reports (home agency forms) originating within the Branch.
p. Consider demobilization well in advance.
q. Debrief with OSC and/or as directed at the end of each shift.
r. Maintain Unit Log (ICS 214-CG).

DIVISION/GROUP SUPERVISOR (DIVS) – The DIVS reports to the OSC (or OPBD when activated). The DIVS is responsible for the implementation of the assigned portion of the IAP, assignment of resources within the Division/Group, and reporting on the progress of control operations and status of resources within the Division/Group.
The major responsibilities of the DIVS are:
a. Review Common Responsibilities in Chapter 2.
b. Obtain briefing from person relieving.
c. Receive briefing from supervisor.
d. Identify resources assigned to the Division/ Group.
e. Provide the IAP to subordinates, as needed.
f. Review Division/Group assigned tasks and incident activities with subordinates.
g. Implement IAP for Division/Group.
h. Supervise Division/Group resources and make changes as appropriate.
i. Ensure through chain of command that Resources Unit is advised of all changes in the status of resources assigned to the Division/ Group.
j. Coordinate activities with adjacent Division/ Group.

7-5

k. Determine need for assistance on assigned tasks.
l. Submit situation and resources status information to the Branch Director or the OSC as directed.
m. Report hazardous situations, special occurrences, or significant events, e.g., accidents, sickness, discovery of unanticipated sensitive resources, to the immediate supervisor.
n. Maintain Unit Log (ICS 214-CG).
o. Ensure that assigned personnel and equipment get to and from assignments in a timely and orderly manner.
p. Resolve logistics problems within the Division/Group.
q. Participate in the development of Branch plans for the next operational period, as requested.
r. Consider demobilization well in advance.
s. Debrief as directed at the end of each shift.
t. Maintain Unit Log (ICS 214-CG).

STRIKE TEAM/TASK FORCE LEADER (STCR/TFLD)

– The STCR/TFLD reports to an OPBD or DIVS and is responsible for performing tactical assignments assigned. The Leader reports work progress, resources status, and other important information and maintains work records on assigned personnel. The major responsibilities of the STCR/TFLD are:
a. Review Common Responsibilities in Chapter 2.
b. Review Common Unit Leader Responsibilities in Chapter 2.
c. Obtain briefing from person you are relieving.
d. Obtain briefing from supervisor.
e. Review assignments with subordinates and assign tasks.
f. Monitor work progress and make changes when necessary.
g. Keep supervisor informed of progress and any changes.

7-6

h. Coordinate activities with adjacent Strike Teams, Task Forces and single resources.
i. Travel to and from active assignment area with assigned resources.
j. Retain control of assigned resources while in available or out-of-service status.
k. Submit situation and resource status information through chain of command DIVS/OPBD/OSC as appropriate.
l. Debrief as directed at the end of each shift.
m. Maintain Unit Log (ICS 214-CG).

SINGLE RESOURCE – The person in charge of a single tactical resource.
The major responsibilities of the Single Resource Leader are:
a. Review Common Responsibilities in Chapter 2.
b. Review assignments.
c. Obtain briefing from person you are relieving.
d. Obtain necessary equipment and supplies.
e. Review weather/environmental conditions for assignment area.
f. Brief subordinates on safety measures.
g. Monitor work progress.
h. Ensure adequate communications with supervisor and subordinates.
i. Keep supervisor informed of progress and any changes.
j. Inform supervisor of problems with assigned resources.
k. Brief relief personnel, and advise them of any change in conditions.
l. Return equipment and supplies to appropriate unit.
m. Complete and turn in all time and use records on personnel and equipment.
n. Debrief as directed at the end of each shift.

   o. Maintain Unit Log (ICS 214-CG).

STAGING AREA MANAGER (STAM) – The STAM is under the direction of the OSC and is responsible for managing all activities within a Staging Area.
The major responsibilities of the STAM are:

   a. Review Common Responsibilities in Chapter 2.

   b. Proceed to Staging Area.

   c. Obtain briefing from person you are relieving.

   d. Establish Staging Area layout.

   e. Determine any support needs for equipment, feeding, sanitation and security.

   f. Establish check-in function as appropriate.

   g. Ensure security of staged resources.

   h. Post areas for identification and traffic control.

   i. Request maintenance service for equipment at Staging Area as appropriate.

   j. Respond to request for resource assignments. (Note: This may be direct from the OSC or via the Incident Communications Center.)

   k. Obtain and issue receipts for radio equipment and other supplies distributed and received at Staging Area.

   l. Determine required resource levels from the OSC.

   m. Advise the OSC when reserve levels reach minimums.

   n. Maintain and provide status to Resource Unit of all resources in Staging Area.

   o. Maintain Staging Area in orderly condition.

   p. Demobilize Staging Area in accordance with the Incident Demobilization Plan.

   q. Debrief with OSC or as directed at the end of each shift.

   r. Maintain Unit Log (ICS 214-CG).

AIR OPERATIONS BRANCH DIRECTOR (AOBD) –

The AOBD is ground-based and is primarily responsible for preparing the Air Operations Summary Worksheet (ICS 220-CG), the air operations portion of the IAP and for providing logistical support to incident aircraft. The Air Operations Summary Worksheet (ICS 220-CG) serves the same purpose as the Work Assignment (ICS 204-CG) does for other operational resources, by assigning and managing aviation resources on the incident. The Air Operations Summary Worksheet (ICS-220-CG) may or may not be completed depending on the needs of the incident. The AOBD will ensure that agency directives, to include Coast Guard Air Operations Manual, COMDTINST M3710.1(series), flight manuals, unit restrictions, and other agency directives will not be violated by incident aircraft, e.g., flight hours, hoist limitations, night flying, etc. Individual aircrews retain primary responsibility to ensure their aircraft are operated in accordance with their own agency's restrictions and directives. It is also the responsibility of individual aircrews to keep the AOBD informed of their agency's restrictions and directives that may affect their ability to execute incident assignments. After the IAP is approved, the AOBD is responsible for overseeing the tactical and logistical assignments of the Air Operations Branch. In coordination with the Logistics Section, the AOBD is responsible for providing logistical support to aircraft operating on the incident.

The major responsibilities of the AOBD are:

    a. Review Common Responsibilities in Chapter 2.

    b. Organize preliminary air operations.

    c. Coordinate airspace use with the FAA. Request declaration (or cancellation) of Temporary Flight Restriction (TFR) IAW FAR 91.173 and post Notice to Airmen (NOTAM) as required.

    d. Attend the tactics meeting and planning meeting to

obtain information for completing the Air Operations Summary Worksheet (ICS 220-CG), if needed.

e. Participate in preparation of the IAP through the OSC. Insure that the air operations portion of the IAP takes into consideration the Air Traffic Control requirements of assigned aircraft.

f. Coordinate with the COML to designate air tactical and support frequencies.

g. Perform operational planning for air operations.

h. Prepare and provide Air Operations Summary Worksheet (ICS 220-CG), if completed, to the Air Support Group and Fixed-Wing Bases.

i. Supervise all air operations activities associated with the incident.

j. Evaluate helibase and helispot locations.

k. Establish procedures for emergency reassignment of aircraft.

l. Coordinate approved flights of non-incident aircraft in the TFR.

m. Coordinate Coast Guard air assets with the appropriate Command Center(s) through normal channels on incident air operations activities.

n. Consider requests for logistical use of incident aircraft.

o. Report to the OSC on air operations activities.

p. Report special incidents/accidents.

q. Develop Aviation Site Safety Plan in concert with SOFR.

r. Arrange for an accident investigation team when warranted.

s. Debrief with OSC as directed at the end of each shift.

t. Maintain Unit Log (ICS 214-CG).

AIR TACTICAL GROUP SUPERVISOR (ATGS) – The ATGS is primarily responsible for tactical operations of

7-10

aircraft and aircrews. This includes: 1) providing fuel and other supplies; 2) providing maintenance and repair of aircraft; 3) keeping records of aircraft activity, and 4) providing enforcement of safety regulations. The ATGS reports to the AOBD.

The major responsibilities of the ATGS are:

    a. Review Common Responsibilities in Chapter 2.

    b. Obtain a copy of the IAP from the AOBD, including Air Operations Summary Worksheet (ICS 220-CG), if completed.

    c. Participate in AOBD planning activities.

    d. Inform AOBD of group activities.

    e. Identify resources/supplies dispatched for the Air Tactical Group.

    f. Request special air tactical items from appropriate sources through Logistics Section.

    g. Coordinate activities with AOBD.

    h. Obtain assigned ground-to-air frequency for airbase operations from the Communications Unit Leader (COML) or Incident Radio Communications Plan (ICS 205-CG).

    i. Inform AOBD of capability to provide night flying service.

    j. Ensure compliance with each agency's operations checklist for day and night operations.

    k. Debrief as directed at the end of each shift.

    l. Maintain Unit Log (ICS 214-CG).

AIR SUPPORT GROUP SUPERVISOR (ASGS) – The ASGS is primarily responsible for supporting aircraft and aircrews. This includes: 1) providing fuel and other supplies; 2) providing maintenance and repair of aircraft; 3) keeping records of aircraft activity, and 4) providing enforcement of safety regulations. The ASGS reports to the AOBD.

The major responsibilities of the ASGS are:

    a. Review Common Responsibilities in Chapter 2.

b. Obtain a copy of the IAP from the AOBD, including Air Operations Summary Worksheet (ICS 220-CG), if completed.

c. Participate in AOBD planning activities.

d. Inform AOBD of group activities.

e. Identify resources/supplies dispatched for the Air Support Group.

f. Request special air support items from appropriate sources through Logistics Section.

g. Determine need for assignment of personnel and equipment at each airbase.

h. Coordinate activities with AOBD.

i. Obtain assigned ground-to-air frequency for airbase operations from the Communications Unit Leader (COML) or Incident Radio Communications Plan (ICS 205-CG).

j. Inform AOBD of capability to provide night flying service.

k. Ensure compliance with each agency's operations checklist for day and night operations.

l. Ensure dust abatement procedures are implemented at helibases and helispots.

m. Provide crash-rescue service for helibases and helispots.

n. Debrief as directed at the end of each shift.

o. Maintain Unit Log (ICS 214-CG).

TECHNICAL SPECIALISTS (THSP) – Certain incidents or events may require the use of THSP's who have specialized knowledge and expertise. THSP's may function within the Planning Section or be assigned wherever their services are required. See chapter 8 and the THSP Job Aid for more detailed information on THSP's.

7-12

CHAPTER 8

PLANNING SECTION

ORGANIZATION CHART

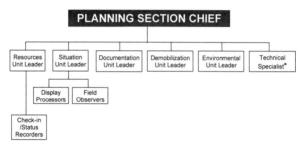

PLANNING SECTION CHIEF

Resources Unit Leader — Situation Unit Leader — Documentation Unit Leader — Demobilization Unit Leader — Environmental Unit Leader — Technical Specialist*

Situation Unit Leader: Display Processors — Field Observers

Resources Unit Leader: Check-in /Status Recorders

* May be assigned wherever their services are required.

References:
- (a) Planning Section Chief Job Aid
- (b) Resource Unit Leader Job Aid
- (c) Situation Unit Leader Job Aid
- (d) Documentation Unit Leader Job Aid
- (e) Demobilization Unit Leader Job Aid
- (f) Environmental Unit Leader Job Aid
- (g) Technical Specialist Job Aid

POSITION CHECKLISTS

PLANNING SECTION CHIEF (PSC) – The PSC, a member of the General Staff, is responsible for the collection, evaluation, dissemination and use of incident information and maintaining status of assigned resources. Information is needed to:
1) Understand the current situation;
2) Predict the probable course of incident events;
3) Prepare strategies, plans and alternative strategies and plans for the incident; and
4) Submit required incident status reports.

The PSC Job Aid, reference (a), should be reviewed regarding the organization and duties of the PSC.

The PSC may have Deputy PSC's, who may be from the same agency or from an assisting agency. The Deputy PSC must have the same qualifications as the person for whom they work, as they must be ready to take over that position at any time.

The major duties of the PSC are:
a. Review Common Responsibilities in Chapter 2.
b. Collect, process, and display incident information.
c. Assist OSC in the development of response strategies.
d. Supervise preparation of the IAP.
e. Facilitate planning meetings and briefings.
f. Supervise the tracking of incident personnel and resources through the Resources Unit.
g. Assign personnel already on-site to ICS organizational positions as appropriate.
h. Establish information requirements and reporting schedules for Planning Section Units (e.g., Resources, Situation).
i. Determine the need for any specialized resources in support of the incident.

8-2

    j. Establish special information collection activities as necessary (e.g., weather, environmental, toxics, etc.).

    k. Assemble information on alternative strategies.

    l. Provide periodic predictions on incident potential.

    m. Keep IMT apprised of any significant changes in incident status.

    n. Compile and display incident status information.

    o. Oversee preparation and implementation of the Incident Demobilization Plan.

    p. Incorporate plans (e.g., Traffic, Medical, Communications, and Site Safety) into the IAP.

    q. Develop other incident supporting plans (e.g., salvage, transition, security).

    r. Review PSC Job Aid.

    s. Maintain Unit Log (ICS 214-CG).

RESOURCE UNIT LEADER (RESL) – The RESL is responsible for maintaining the status of all assigned tactical resources and personnel at an incident. This is achieved by overseeing the check-in of all tactical resources and personnel, maintaining a status-keeping system indicating current location and status of all these resources. The RESL Job Aid, Reference (b), should be reviewed regarding the organization and duties of the RESL.

The major responsibilities of the RESL are:

    a. Review Common Responsibilities in Chapter 2.

    b. Review Unit Leader Responsibilities in Chapter 2.

    c. Establish the check-in function at incident locations.

    d. Prepare Organization Assignment List (ICS 203-CG) and Organization Chart (ICS 207-CG).

    e. Prepare appropriate parts of Division Assignment Lists (ICS 204-CG).

    f. Maintain and post the current status and location of all tactical resources.

8-3

g. Maintain master roster of all tactical resources checked in at the incident.
h. Attend meetings and briefings as required by the PSC.
i. Review Resource Unit Leader Job Aid.
j. Maintain Unit Log (ICS 214-CG).

CHECK-IN/STATUS RECORDER (SCKN) – SCKN's are needed at each check-in location to ensure that all resources assigned to an incident are accounted for. The major responsibilities of the SCKN are:

a. Review Common Responsibilities in Chapter 2.
b. Obtain required work materials, including Check-in Lists (ICS 211-CG), Resource Status Cards (ICS-219) and status display boards or T-card racks.
c. Post signs so that arriving resources can easily find incident check-in location(s).
d. Record check-in information on Check-in Lists (ICS 211-CG).
e. Transmit check-in information to the RESL.
f. Forward completed ICS 211-CG and Status Change Cards (ICS-210) to the RESL.
g. Receive, record, and maintain resource status information on Resource Status Cards (ICS-219) for incident-assigned tactical resources, and overhead personnel.
h. Maintain files of Check-in Lists (ICS 211-CG).
i. Maintain Unit Log (ICS 214-CG).

SITUATION UNIT LEADER (SITL) – The Situation Unit Leader is responsible for collecting, processing and organizing incident information relating to the growth, mitigation or intelligence activities taking place on the incident. The SITL may prepare future projections of incident growth, maps and intelligence information. The

SITL Job Aid, reference (c), should be reviewed regarding the organization and duties of the SITL. The major responsibilities of the SITL are:

a. Review Common Responsibilities in Chapter 2.
b. Review Unit Leader Responsibilities in Chapter 2.
c. Begin collection and analysis of incident data as soon as possible.
d. Prepare, post, or disseminate resource and situation status information as required, including special requests.
e. Prepare periodic predictions or as requested by the PSC.
f. Prepare the Incident Status Summary Form (ICS 209-CG).
g. Provide photographic services and maps if required.
h. Conduct situation briefings at meetings and briefings as required by the PSC.
i. Develop and maintain master chart(s)/map(s) of the incident.
j. Maintain chart/map of incident in the common area of the ICP for all responders to view.
k. Maintain Unit Log (ICS 214-CG).

DISPLAY PROCESSOR (DPRO) – The DPRO is responsible for the display of incident status information obtained from Field Observers (FOBS), resource status reports, aerial and other photographs, and infrared data.

The major responsibilities of the DPRO are:

a. Review Common Responsibilities in Chapter 2.
b. Determine:
   - Location of work assignment
   - Numbers, types and locations of displays required
   - Priorities

8-5

- Map requirements for the IAP
- Time limits for completion

c. Obtain necessary equipment and supplies.

d. Assist SITL in analyzing and evaluating field reports.

e. Develop required displays in accordance with time limits for completion. Examples of displays include:
  - GIS information
  - Demographic information
  - Incident projection data
  - Enlargement of ICS forms

f. Maintain Unit Log (ICS 214-CG).

FIELD OBSERVER (FOBS) – The FOBS is responsible for collecting situation information from personal observations at the incident and provides this information to the SITL. The major responsibilities of the FOBS are:

a. Review Common Responsibilities in Chapter 2.

b. Determine:
  - Location of assignment
  - Type of information required
  - Priorities
  - Time limits for completion
  - Method of communication
  - Method of transportation

c. Obtain necessary equipment and supplies.

d. Perform FOBS responsibilities to include but not limited to the following:
  - Perimeters of incident
  - Locations of trouble spots
  - Weather conditions
  - Hazards
  - Progress of operations resources

e. Be prepared to identify all facility locations (e.g.,

8-6

Helispots, Division and Branch boundaries).

f.   Report information to the SITL by established procedure.
g.   Report immediately any condition observed that may cause danger and a safety hazard to personnel.
h.   Gather intelligence that will lead to accurate predictions.
i.   Maintain Unit Log (ICS 214-CG).

DOCUMENTATION UNIT LEADER (DOCL) – The DOCL is responsible for the maintenance of accurate, up-to-date incident files. Examples of incident documentation include: Incident Action Plan(s), incident reports, communication logs, injury claims, situation status reports, etc. Thorough documentation is critical to post-incident analysis. Some of the documents may originate in other sections. The DOCL shall ensure each section is maintaining and providing appropriate documents. The DOCL will provide duplication and copying services for all other sections. The Documentation Unit will store incident files for legal, analytical, and historical purposes. The DOCL Job Aid, reference (d), should be reviewed regarding the organization and duties of the DOCL.
The major responsibilities of the DOCL are:

a.   Review Common Responsibilities in Chapter 2.
b.   Review Unit Leader Responsibilities in Chapter 2.
c.   Set up work area; begin organization of incident files.
d.   Establish duplication service; respond to requests.
e.   File all official forms and reports.
f.   Review records for accuracy and completeness; inform appropriate units of errors or omissions.
g.   Provide incident documentation as requested.
h.   Organize files for submitting final incident

documentation package.
i. Maintain Unit Log (ICS 214-CG).

DEMOBILIZATION UNIT LEADER (DMOB) – The

DMOB is responsible for developing the Incident Demobilization Plan. On large incidents, demobilization can be quite complex, requiring a separate planning activity. Note that not all agencies require specific demobilization instructions. The DMOB Job Aid, reference (e), should be reviewed regarding the organization and duties of the DMOB.
The major responsibilities of the DMOB are:

a. Review Common Responsibilities in Chapter 2.
b. Review Unit Leader Responsibilities in Chapter 2.
c. Review incident resource records to determine the likely size and extent of demobilization effort and develop a resource matrix.
d. Coordinate demobilization with Agency Representatives.
e. Monitor the on-going Operations Section resource needs.
f. Identify surplus resources and probable release time.
g. Establish communications with off-incident facilities, as necessary.
h. Develop an Incident Demobilization Plan that should include:
   • General information section
   • Responsibilities section
   • Release priorities
   • Release procedures
   • Demobilization Checkout Form (ICS-221-CG)
   • Directory
i. Prepare appropriate directories (e.g., maps, instructions, etc.) for inclusion in the demobilization plan.

    j.   Distribute demobilization plan (on and off-site).
    k.   Provide status reports to appropriate requestors.
    l.   Ensure that all Sections/Units understand their specific demobilization responsibilities.
    m. Supervise execution of the Incident Demobilization Plan.
    n.   Brief the PSC on demobilization progress.
    o.   Review DMOB Job Aid.
    p.   Maintain Unit Log (ICS 214-CG).

The following are examples of optional Unit Leader positions that can be established and used as needed during an incident:

ENVIRONMENTAL UNIT LEADER (ENVL) – The ENVL is responsible for environmental matters associated with the response, including strategic assessment, modeling, surveillance, and environmental monitoring and permitting. The ENVL prepares environmental data for the Situation Unit. Technical Specialists frequently assigned to the Environmental Unit may include the Scientific Support Coordinator and Sampling, Response Technologies, Trajectory Analysis, Weather Forecast, Resources at Risk, Shoreline Cleanup Assessment, Historical/ Cultural Resources, and Disposal Technical Specialists. The ENVL Job Aid, reference (f), should be reviewed regarding the organization and duties of the ENVL.
The major responsibilities of the ENVL are:
    a.   Review Common Responsibilities in Chapter 2.
    b.   Review Unit Leader Responsibilities in Chapter 2.
    c.   Obtain a briefing and special instructions from the PSC.
    d.   Identify sensitive areas and recommend response priorities.
    e.   Following consultation with natural resource trustees, provide input on wildlife protection

8-9

strategies (e.g., removing oiled carcasses, pre-emptive capture, hazing, and/or capture and treatment).

f. Determine the extent, fate, and effects of contamination.

g. Acquire, distribute, and provide analysis of weather forecasts.

h. Monitor the environmental consequences of response actions.

i. Develop shoreline cleanup and assessment plans. Identify the need for, and prepare any special advisories or orders.

j. Identify the need for, and obtain, permits, consultations, and other authorizations, including Endangered Species Act (ESA) provisions.

k. Following consultation with the FOSC's Historical/Cultural Resources Technical Specialist identify and develop plans for protection of affected historical/cultural resources.

l. Evaluate the opportunities to use various response technologies.

m. Develop disposal plans.

n. Develop a plan for collecting, transporting, and analyzing samples.

o. Review ENVL Job Aid.

p. Maintain Unit Log (ICS 214-CG).

MARINE TRANSPORTATION SYSTEM RECOVERY UNIT LEADER (MTSL) – The MTSL is responsible for planning infrastructure recovery for Transportation Security Incidents (TSI) (see chapter 16) and other incidents that significantly impact the Marine Transportation System (MTS). The MTSL will track and report on the status of the MTS, understand critical recovery pathways, recommend courses of action, and provide all MTS stakeholders with an avenue of input to the response organization. The MTSL prepares transportation data for the Situation Unit and daily situation briefs applying core Essential Elements of Information (EEIs). Sample EEIs include Deep draft shipping, Aids to Navigation, Bulk liquid facilities, Intermodal connections, Bridges, Vessel Salvage, etc. The major responsibilities of the MTSL are:

a. Review Common Responsibilities in Chapter 2.

b. Review Unit Leader Responsibilities in Chapter 2.

c. Obtain a briefing and special instructions from the PSC.

d. Support Operation Section Staff elements that are established for MTS Recovery.

e. Identify, track and report impacts to the MTS in accordance with EEIs.

f. Coordinate and consult with MTS stakeholders. Solicit periodic and standardized feedback from impacted industries/stakeholders.

g. Identify resources, agencies involved, and courses of action for the recovery of public infrastructure such as ATON, communications systems, and federal channels.

h. Prioritize recovery operations (including ATON, dredging, salvage, cleanup, repair, etc), as appropriate.

i. Monitor the economic consequences of recovery actions.

j. Develop traffic management plans. Identify the need for, and prepare any special advisories or orders (i.e. Safety/Security Zone).

k. Assess the need for MTS relief measures outside the impacted area. Implement measures (i.e. redirect cargos, establish alternate transportation modes) as necessary.

l. Liaise with MTS Response Branch Director (TRBD) to execute operational objectives.

m. Maintain Unit Log (ICS 214-CG).

INTELLIGENCE UNIT LEADER (IUL) – See Chapter 11.

TECHNICAL SPECIALISTS (THSP) – Certain incidents or events may require the use of THSP's who have specialized knowledge and expertise. THSP's may function within the Planning Section or be assigned wherever their services are required. The THSP Job Aid, reference (g), should be reviewed for more detailed information. The major responsibilities of the THSP are:

   a. Review Common Responsibilities in Chapter 2.
   b. Provide technical expertise and advice to Command and General Staff as needed.
   c. Attend meetings and briefings as appropriate to clarify and help to resolve technical issues within area of expertise.
   d. Maintain Unit Log (ICS 214-CG).

Other major responsibilities that might apply to the THSP as appropriate:

   e. Provide technical expertise during the development of the IAP and other support plans.
   f. Work with the Safety Officer to mitigate unsafe practices.
   g. Work closely with Liaison Officer to help facilitate understanding among stakeholders and special interest groups.
   h. Be available to attend press briefings to clarify technical issues.
   i. Research technical issues and provide findings to decision makers.
   j. Trouble shoot technical problems and provide advice on resolution.
   k. Review specialized plans and clarify meaning.

The following are examples of Technical Specialists. This is not a complete list but examples of the many kinds of THSP's that may be used with a possible location for the position in the ICS organization. However, <u>the IC may assign THSP's to any location within the ICS organization based on incident need</u>. For example, the CISM Specialist is normally assigned in Logistics under the Medical Unit Leader; however, an additional CISM Specialist is often assigned in the Command Staff working directly for the IC. Please see the THSP job aid for more information on each of the positions.

Command Staff:
- Auxiliary Liaison Specialist
- Legal specialist
- Volunteer Specialist/Coordinator

Operations:
- Air Tanker/Fixed Wing Coordinator
- Helicopter Coordinator
- Helibase Manager
- Helispot Manager

Planning:
- Documentation Specialist
- Environmental Specialist
- Geographic Information System Specialist
- Historian
- Public Health Specialist
- Salvage and Engineering Technical Specialist
- Situation Report Specialist
- Training Specialist
- Weather Observer

Logistics:
- Berthing Manager
- Camp Manager
- Cashier Manager
- Communications Restoration Manager
- Contingency Communications Manager

- Chaplain
- Critical Incident Stress Management (CISM) Specialist/Coordinator
- Damage Assessment Teams
- Evacuation Teams/Specialists
- Entitlement Specialist
- Facility Repair and Reconstruction Manager
- Facility Maintenance/Repair Teams/Specialists
- Family Assistance Specialist/Coordinator
- Food Teams/Specialists
- Human Resource Specialist
- Receiving and Distribution Manager
- Legal Support Teams/Specialists
- Medical Teams/Specialists
- Personnel Accountability Manager
- Personnel Support Teams/Specialists

CHAPTER 9

LOGISTICS SECTION

ORGANIZATION CHART

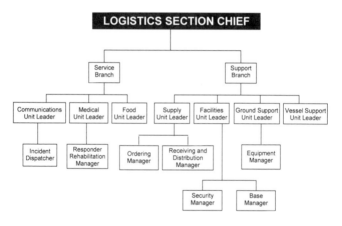

Reference:
  (a) Logistics Section Chief Job Aid

POSITION CHECKLISTS

LOGISTICS SECTION CHIEF (LSC) – The LSC, a member of the General Staff, is responsible for providing facilities, services, and material in support of the incident. The LSC participates in the development and implementation of the IAP and activates and supervises the Branches and Units within the Logistics Section. The LSC Job Aid, reference (a), should be reviewed regarding the organization and duties of the LSC.

The LSC may have Deputy LSC's, who may be from the same agency or from an assisting agency. The Deputy LSC must have the same qualifications as the person for whom they work, as they must be ready to take over that position at any time.

The major responsibilities of the LSC are:
   a. Review Common Responsibilities in Chapter 2.
   b. Plan the organization of the Logistics Section.
   c. Assign work locations and preliminary work tasks to Section personnel.
   d. Notify the Resources Unit of the Logistics Section Units activated, including names and locations of assigned personnel.
   e. Assemble and brief Logistics Branch Directors and Unit Leaders.
   f. Determine and supply immediate incident resource and facility needs.
   g. In conjunction with Command, develop and advise all Sections of the IMT resource approval and requesting process.
   h. Review proposed tactics for upcoming operational period for ability to provide resources and logistical support.
   i. Identify long-term service and support

9-2

requirements for planned and expected operations.

j. Advise Command and other Section Chiefs on resource availability to support incident needs.

k. Provide input to and review the Communications Plan, Medical Plan and Traffic Plan.

l. Identify resource needs for incident contingencies.

m. Coordinate and process requests for additional resources.

n. Track resource effectiveness and make necessary adjustments.

o. Advise on current service and support capabilities.

p. Request and/or set up expanded ordering processes as appropriate to support incident.

q. Develop recommended list of Section resources to be demobed and initiate recommendation for release when appropriate.

r. Receive and implement applicable portions of the incident Demobilization Plan.

s. Ensure the general welfare and safety of Logistics Section personnel.

t. Maintain Unit Log (ICS 214-CG).

SERVICE BRANCH DIRECTOR (SVBD) – The SVBD, when activated, is under the supervision of the LSC and is responsible for the management of all service activities at the incident. The Branch Director supervises the operations of the Communications, Medical and Food Units.

The major responsibilities of the SVBD are:

a. Review Common Responsibilities in Chapter 2.

b. Review Unit Leader Responsibilities in Chapter 2.

c. Obtain working materials.

d. Determine the level of service required to support operations.

9-3

e. Confirm dispatch of Branch personnel.
f. Participate in planning meetings of Logistics Section personnel.
g. Review the IAP.
h. Organize and prepare assignments for Service Branch personnel.
i. Coordinate activities of Branch Units.
j. Inform the LSC of Branch activities.
k. Resolve Service Branch problems.
l. Maintain Unit Log (ICS 214-CG).

COMMUNICATIONS UNIT LEADER (COML) – The COML is responsible for developing plans for the effective use of incident communications equipment and facilities; installing and testing of communications equipment; supervision of the Incident Communications Center; distribution of communications equipment to incident personnel; and the maintenance and repair of communications equipment.

The major responsibilities of the COML are:
a. Review Common Responsibilities in Chapter 2.
b. Review Unit Leader Responsibilities in Chapter 2.
c. Determine Unit personnel needs.
d. Prepare and implement the Incident Radio Communications Plan (ICS 205-CG).
e. Ensure the Incident Communications Center and the Message Center is established.
f. Establish appropriate communications distribution/maintenance locations within the Base.
g. Ensure communications systems are installed and tested.
h. Ensure an equipment accountability system is established.
i. Ensure personal portable radio equipment from cache is distributed per Incident Radio Communications Plan.

9-4

   j. Provide technical information as required on:
- Adequacy of communications systems currently in operation.
- Geographic limitation on communications systems.
- Equipment capabilities/limitations.
- Amount and types of equipment available.
- Anticipated problems in the use of communications equipment.

   k. Supervise Communications Unit activities.

   l. Maintain records on all communications equipment as appropriate.

  m. Ensure equipment is tested and repaired.

   n. Recover equipment from Units being demobilized.

   o. Maintain Unit Log (ICS 214-CG).

INCIDENT DISPATCHER (INCM) – The INCM is responsible for receiving and transmitting radio and telephone messages among and between personnel and to provide dispatch services at the incident. The major responsibilities of the INCM are:

   a. Review Common Responsibilities in Chapter 2.

   b. Ensure adequate staffing.

   c. Obtain and review the IAP to determine the incident organization and Incident Radio Communications Plan.

   d. Set up Incident Radio Communications Center; check-out equipment.

   e. Request service on any inoperable or marginal equipment.

   f. Set-up Message Center location, as required.

   g. Receive and transmit messages within and external to the incident.

   h. Maintain files of ICS-210 and General Messages (ICS 213-CG).

   i. Maintain a record of unusual incident

occurrences.

j. Provide a briefing to relief personnel on:
   - Current activities.
   - Equipment status.
   - Any unusual communications situations.
k. Turn in appropriate documents to the Communications Unit Leader.
l. Demobilize the Communications Center in accordance with the Incident Demobilization Plan.
m. Maintain Unit Log (ICS 214-CG).

MEDICAL UNIT LEADER (MEDL) – The MEDL, under the direction of the Service Branch Director or Logistics Section Chief, is primarily responsible for the development of the Medical Plan; providing medical care and overseeing health aspects of response personnel; obtaining medical aid and transportation for injured and ill response personnel; coordinating with other functions to resolve heath and safety issues; and preparation of reports and records.
The major responsibilities of the MEDL are:

a. Review Common Responsibilities in Chapter 2.
b. Review Unit Leader Responsibilities in Chapter 2.
c. Participate in Logistics Section/Service Branch planning activities.
d. Establish the Medical Unit.
e. Prepare the Medical Plan (ICS 206-CG).
f. Provide any relevant medical input into the planning process for strategy development.
g. Coordinate with Safety Officer, Operations, hazmat specialists, and others on proper personnel protection procedures for incident personnel.
h. Prepare procedures for major medical emergency.
i. Develop transportation routes and methods for

injured incident personnel.

j. Ensure incident personnel patients are tracked as they move from origin, care facility and disposition.

k. Provide continuity of medical care for incident personnel.

l. Declare major medical emergency as appropriate.

m. Provide or oversee medical and rehab care delivered to incident personnel.

n. Monitor health aspects of incident personnel including excessive incident stress.

o. Respond to requests for medical aid, medical transportation and medical supplies.

p. In conjunction with Finance/Admin Section, prepare and submit necessary authorizations, reports and administrative documentation related to injuries, compensation or death of incident personnel.

q. Coordinate personnel and mortuary affairs for incident personnel fatalities.

r. Provide oversight and liaison as necessary for incident victims among emergency medical care, medical examiner and hospital care.

s. Provide for security and proper disposition of incident medical records.

t. Maintain Unit Log (ICS 214-CG).

RESPONDER REHABILITATION MANAGER (REHB)
– The REHB reports to the Medical Unit Leader and is responsible for the rehabilitation of incident personnel who are suffering from the effects of strenuous work and/or extreme conditions.

The major responsibilities of the REHB are:

a. Review Common Responsibilities in Chapter 2.

b. Designate the responder rehabilitation location and have the location announced on the radio with radio designation "Rehab".

9-7

c. Coordinate with MEDL to request necessary medical personnel to evaluate the medical condition of personnel being rehabilitated.
d. Request necessary resources for rehabilitation of personnel, e.g., water, juice, personnel.
e. Request food through the Food Unit or LSC, as necessary, for personnel being rehabilitated.
f. Release rehabilitated personnel for reassignment.
g. Maintain appropriate records and documentation.
h. Maintain Unit Log (ICS 214-CG).

FOOD UNIT LEADER (FDUL) – The FDUL is responsible for supplying the food needs for the entire incident, including all remote locations, e.g., Staging Areas, as well as providing food for personnel unable to leave tactical field assignments.
The major responsibilities of the FDUL are:
a. Review Common Responsibilities in Chapter 2.
b. Review Unit Leader Responsibilities in Chapter 2.
c. Determine food and water requirements.
d. Determine the method of feeding to best fit each facility or situation.
e. Obtain necessary equipment and supplies.
f. Ensure that well-balanced menus are provided.
g. Order sufficient food and potable water from the Supply Unit.
h. Maintain an inventory of food and water.
i. Maintain food service areas, ensuring that all appropriate health and safety measures are being followed.
j. Supervise Food Unit personnel as appropriate.
k. Maintain Unit Log (ICS 214-CG).

SUPPORT BRANCH DIRECTOR (SUBD) – The SUBD, when activated, is under the direction of the LSC, and is responsible for the development and implementation of logistics plans in support of the

9-8

Incident Action Plan. The SUBD supervises the operations of the Supply, Facilities, Ground Support and Vessel Support Units.

The major responsibilities of the SUBD are:

a. Review Common Responsibilities in Chapter 2
b. Review Unit Leader Responsibilities in Chapter 2.
c. Obtain work materials.
d. Identify Support Branch personnel dispatched to the incident.
e. Determine initial support operations in coordination with the LSC and SVBD.
f. Prepare initial organization and assignments for support operations.
g. Assemble and brief Support Branch personnel.
h. Determine if assigned Branch resources are sufficient.
i. Maintain surveillance of assigned Units work progress and inform the LSC of their activities.
j. Resolve problems associated with requests from the Operations Section.
k. Maintain Unit Log (ICS 214-CG).

SUPPLY UNIT LEADER (SPUL) – The SPUL is primarily responsible for receiving, storing and distributing all supplies for the incident; maintaining an inventory of supplies; and storing, disbursing and servicing non-expendable supplies and equipment.

The major responsibilities of the SPUL are:

a. Review Common Responsibilities in Chapter 2.
b. Review Unit Leader Responsibilities in Chapter 2.
c. Participate in Logistics Section/Support Branch planning activities.
d. Determine the type and amount of supplies enroute.
e. Review the IAP for information on operations of the Supply Unit.
f. Develop and implement safety and security

9-9

requirements.

g. Order, receive, distribute and store supplies and equipment.
h. Receive and respond to requests for personnel, supplies and equipment.
i. Maintain an inventory of supplies and equipment.
j. Service reusable equipment.
k. Submit reports to the SUBD.
l. Maintain Unit Log (ICS 214-CG).

ORDERING MANAGER (ORDM) – The ORDM is responsible for placing all orders for supplies and equipment for the incident. The ORDM reports to the SPUL. The major responsibilities of the ORDM are:

a. Review Common Responsibilities in Chapter 2.
b. Obtain necessary agency(s) order forms.
c. Establish ordering procedures.
d. Establish name and telephone numbers of agency(s) personnel receiving orders.
e. Set up filing system.
f. Obtain roster of incident personnel who have ordering authority.
g. Obtain list of previously ordered supplies and equipment.
h. Ensure order forms are filled out correctly.
i. Place orders in a timely manner.
j. Consolidate orders, when possible.
k. Identify times and locations for delivery of supplies and equipment.
l. Keep RCDM informed of orders placed.
m. Submit all ordering documents to the Documentation Control Unit through the SPUL Leader before demobilization.
n. Maintain Unit Log (ICS 214-CG).

RECEIVING AND DISTRIBUTION MANAGER (RCDM) – The RCDM is responsible for receiving and

9-10

distributing all supplies and equipment (other than primary resources) and the service and repair of tools and equipment. The RCDM reports to the SPUL.
The major responsibilities of the RCDM are:

    a. Review Common Responsibilities in Chapter 2.
    b. Order required personnel to operate supply area.
    c. Organize the physical layout of the supply area.
    d. Establish procedures for operating the supply area.
    e. Set up a filing system for receiving and distributing supplies and equipment.
    f. Maintain inventory of supplies and equipment.
    g. Develop security requirement for supply area.
    h. Establish procedures for receiving supplies and equipment.
    i. Submit necessary reports to the SPUL.
    j. Notify ORDM of supplies and equipment received.
    k. Provide necessary supply records to SPUL. Leader.
    l. Maintain Unit Log (ICS 214-CG).

FACILITIES UNIT LEADER (FACL) – The FACL is primarily responsible for the set up, maintenance and demobilization of incident facilities, e.g., Base, ICP and Staging Areas, as well as security services required to support incident operations. The FACL provides sleeping and sanitation facilities for incident personnel and manages Base operations. Each facility is assigned a manager who reports to the FACL and is responsible for managing the operation of the facility. The FACL reports to the SUBD.
The major responsibilities of the FACL are:

    a. Review Common Responsibilities in Chapter 2.
    b. Review Unit Leader Responsibilities in Chapter 2.
    c. Obtain a briefing from the SUBD or the LSC.
    d. Receive and review a copy of the IAP.

e. Participate in Logistics Section/Support Branch planning activities.
f. In conjunction with the Finance/Admin Section, determine locations suitable for incident support facilities and secure permission to use through appropriate means.
g. Inspect facilities prior to occupation and document conditions and preexisting damage.
h. Determine requirements for each facility, including the ICP.
i. Prepare layouts of incident facilities.
j. Notify Unit Leaders of facility layout.
k. Activate incident facilities.
j. Provide Facility Managers and personnel to operate facilities.
k. Provide sleeping facilities.
l. Provide security services.
m. Provide food and water service.
n. Provide sanitation and shower service, as needed.
o. Provide facility maintenance services, e.g., sanitation, lighting, clean up, trash removal, etc.
p. Inspect all facilities for damage and potential claims.
q. Demobilize incident facilities.
r. Maintain facility records.
s. Maintain Unit Log (ICS 214-CG).

SECURITY MANAGER (SECM) – The SECM is responsible for providing safeguards needed to protect personnel and property from loss or damage.
The major responsibilities of the SECM are:
a. Review Common Responsibilities in Chapter 2.
b. Establish contacts with local law enforcement agencies, as required.
c. Contact the Resource Use Specialist for crews or Agency Representatives to discuss any special

custodial requirements that may affect operations.
d. Request required personnel support to accomplish work assignments.
e. Ensure security of classified material and/or systems.
f. Ensure that support personnel are qualified to manage security problems.
g. Develop Security Plan for incident facilities.
h. Adjust Security Plan for personnel and equipment changes and releases.
i. Coordinate security activities with appropriate incident personnel.
j. Keep the peace, prevent assaults and settle disputes through coordination with Agency Representatives.
k. Prevent theft of all government and personal property.
l. Document all complaints and suspicious occurrences.
m. Maintain Unit Log (ICS 214-CG).

BASE MANAGER (BCMG) – The BCMG is responsible for ensuring that appropriate sanitation, security and facility management services are conducted at the Base. The major responsibilities of the BCMG are:
a. Review Common Responsibilities in Chapter 2.
b. Determine personnel support requirements.
c. Obtain necessary equipment and supplies.
d. Ensure that all facilities and equipment are set up and properly functioning.
e. Supervise the establishment of
  • Sanitation facilities, including showers, and
  • Sleeping facilities.
f. Make sleeping area assignments.
g. Adhere to all applicable safety and health standards and regulations.
h. Ensure that all facility maintenance services are

9-13

provided.
i.   Maintain Unit Log (ICS 214-CG).

GROUND SUPPORT UNIT LEADER (GSUL) – The
GSUL is primarily responsible for ensuring: repair of
primary tactical equipment, vehicles, mobile ground
support equipment and fueling services; transportation
of personnel, supplies, food and equipment in support
of incident operations; recording all ground equipment
usage time, including contract equipment assigned to
the incident; and implementing the Traffic Plan for the
incident. The major responsibilities of the GSUL are:
a.   Review Common Responsibilities in Chapter 2.
b.   Review Unit Leader Responsibilities in Chapter 2.
c.   Participate in Support Branch/Logistics Section
     planning activities.
d.   Develop and implement the Traffic Plan.
e.   Support out-of-service resources.
f.   Notify the Resources Unit of all status changes on
     support and transportation vehicles.
g.   Arrange for and activate fueling, maintenance and
     repair of ground resources.
h.   Maintain Support Vehicle Inventory and
     transportation vehicles (ICS-218).
i.   Provide transportation services IAW requests
     from the LSC or SUBD.
j.   Collect use information on rented equipment.
k.   Requisition maintenance and repair supplies,
     e.g., fuel, spare parts.
l.   Maintain incident roads.
m.   Submit reports to SUBD as directed.
n.   Maintain Unit Log (ICS 214-CG).

EQUIPMENT MANAGER (EQPM) – The EQPM
provides service, repair and fuel for all apparatus and
equipment; provides transportation and support vehicle
services; and maintains records of equipment use and

service provided.

The major responsibilities of the EQPM are:

- a. Review Common Responsibilities in Chapter 2.
- b. Obtain the IAP to determine locations for assigned resources, Staging Area locations and fueling and service requirements for all resources.
- c. Obtain necessary equipment and supplies.
- d. Provide maintenance and fueling according to schedule.
- e. Prepare schedules to maximize use of available transportation.
- f. Provide transportation and support vehicles for incident use.
- g. Coordinate with AREP on service and repair policies, as required.
- h. Inspect equipment condition and ensure coverage by equipment agreement.
- i. Determine supplies (e.g., gasoline, diesel, oil and parts needed to maintain equipment in an efficient operating condition) and place orders with the Supply Unit.
- j. Maintain Support Vehicle Inventory (ICS-218).
- k. Maintain equipment rental records.
- l. Maintain equipment service and use records.
- m. Check all service repair areas to ensure that all appropriate safety measures are being taken.
- n. Maintain Unit Log (ICS 214-CG).

VESSEL SUPPORT UNIT LEADER (VESS) – The VESS is responsible for implementing the Vessel Routing Plan for the incident and coordinating transportation on the water and between shore resources. Since most vessels will be supported by their own infrastructure, the Vessel Support Unit may be requested to arrange fueling, dockage, maintenance and repair of vessels on a case-by-case basis.

The major responsibilities of the VESS are:

a. Review Common Responsibilities in Chapter 2.

b. Review Unit Leader Responsibilities in Chapter 2.

c. Obtain a briefing from the SUBD or the LSC.

d. Participate in Support Branch/Logistics Section planning activities.

e. Coordinate development of the Vessel Routing Plan.

f. Coordinate vessel transportation assignments with the Protection and Recovery Branch or other sources of vessel transportation.

g. Coordinate water-to-land transportation with the Ground Support Unit, as necessary.

h. Maintain a prioritized list of transportation requirements that need to be scheduled with the transportation source.

i. Support out-of-service vessel resources, as requested.

j. Arrange for fueling, dockage, maintenance and repair of vessel resources, as requested.

k. Maintain inventory of support and transportation vessels.

l. Maintain Unit Log (ICS 214-CG).

TECHNICAL SPECIALISTS (THSP) – Certain incidents or events may require the use of THSP's who have specialized knowledge and expertise. THSP's may function within the Planning Section or be assigned wherever their services are required. See chapter 8 and the THSP Job Aid for more detailed information on THSP's.

CHAPTER 10

FINANCE/ADMINISTRATION SECTION

ORGANIZATION CHART

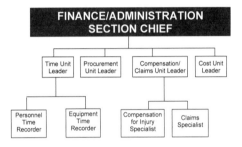

Reference:
   (a) Finance/Administration Section Chief Job Aid

POSITION CHECKLISTS

FINANCE/ADMINISTRATION SECTION CHIEF (FSC)

- The FSC, a member of the General Staff, is responsible for all financial, administrative and cost analysis aspects of the incident and for supervising members of the Finance/Admin Section. The FSC Job Aid (reference (a)) should be reviewed regarding the organization and duties of the FSC.

The FSC may have Deputy FSC's, who may be from the same agency or from an assisting agency. The Deputy FSC must have the same qualifications as the person for whom they work, as they must be ready to take over that position at any time.

The major responsibilities of the FSC are:

a. Review Common Responsibilities in Chapter 2.
b. Participate in incident planning meetings and briefings as required.
c. Review operational plans and provide alternatives where financially appropriate.
d. Manage all financial aspects of an incident.
e. Provide financial and cost analysis information as requested.
f. Gather pertinent information from briefings with responsible agencies.
g. Develop an operating plan for the Finance/ Admin Section; fill supply and support needs.
h. Determine the need to set up and operate an incident commissary.
i. Meet with Assisting and Cooperating Agency Representatives, as needed.
j. Maintain daily contact with agency(s) administrative headquarters on Finance/Admin matters.
k. Ensure that all personnel time records are

10-2

accurately completed and transmitted to home agencies, according to policy.

l. Provide financial input to demobilization planning.

m. Ensure that all obligation documents initiated at the incident are properly prepared and completed.

n. Brief agency administrative personnel on all incident-related financial issues needing attention or follow-up prior to leaving incident.

o. Develop recommended list of Section resources to be demobed and initial recommendation for release when appropriate.

p. Receive and implement applicable portions of the incident Demobilization Plan.

q. Maintain Unit Log (ICS 214-CG).

TIME UNIT LEADER (TIME) - The TIME is responsible for equipment and personnel time recording and for managing the commissary operations.

The major responsibilities of the TIME are:

a. Review Common Responsibilities in Chapter 2.

b. Review Unit Leader Responsibilities in Chapter 2.

c. Determine incident requirements for time recording function.

d. Determine resource needs.

e. Contact appropriate agency personnel/ representatives.

f. Ensure that daily personnel time recording documents are prepared and in compliance with agency(s) policy.

g. Establish time unit objectives.

h. Maintain separate logs for overtime hours.

i. Establish commissary operation on larger or long-term incidents, as needed.

j. Submit cost estimate data forms to the Cost Unit, as required.

k. Maintain records security.

   l. Ensure that all records are current and complete prior to demobilization.

   m. Release time reports from assisting agency personnel to the respective Agency Representatives prior to demobilization.

   n. Brief the FSC on current problems and recommendations, outstanding issues and follow-up requirements.

   o. Maintain Unit Log (ICS 214-CG).

EQUIPMENT TIME RECORDER (EQTR) - Under supervision of the TIME, the EQTR is responsible for overseeing the recording of time for all equipment assigned to an incident.

The major responsibilities of the EQTR are:

   a. Review Common Responsibilities in Chapter 2.

   b. Set up the EQTR function in location designated by the Time Unit Leader.

   c. Advise Ground Support Unit, Vessel Support Unit, Facilities Unit and Air Support Group of the requirement to establish and maintain a file for maintaining a daily record of equipment time.

   d. Assist Units in establishing a system for collecting equipment time reports.

   e. Post all equipment time tickets within 4 hours after the end of each operational period.

   f. Prepare a use and summary invoice for equipment, as required, within 12 hours after equipment arrival at the incident.

   g. Submit data to TIME for cost effectiveness analysis.

   h. Maintain current posting on all charges or credits for fuel, parts and services.

   i. Verify all time data and deductions with owner/operator of equipment.

   j. Complete all forms according to agency specifications.

    k.   Close out forms prior to demobilization.
    l.   Distribute copies per agency and incident policy.
    m. Maintain Unit Log (ICS 214-CG).

PERSONNEL TIME RECORDER (PTRC) - Under supervision of the TIME, the PTRC is responsible for overseeing the recording of time for all personnel assigned to an incident.
The major responsibilities of the PTRC are:
    a. Review Common Responsibilities in Chapter 2.
    b. Establish and maintain a file for incident personnel time reports within the first operational period.
    c. Initiate, gather or update a time report from all applicable personnel assigned to the incident for each operational period.
    d. Ensure that all employee identification information is verified to be correct on the time report.
    e. Post personnel travel and work hours, transfers, promotions, specific pay provisions and terminations to personnel time documents.
    f. Ensure that time reports are signed.
    g. Close-out time documents prior to personnel leaving the incident.
    h. Distribute all time documents according to agency policy.
    i. Maintain a log of excessive hours worked and give to the TIME daily.
    j. Maintain Unit Log (ICS 214-CG).

PROCUREMENT UNIT LEADER (PROC) - The PROC is responsible for administering all financial matters pertaining to vendor contracts, leases and fiscal agreements.
The major responsibilities of the PROC are:
    a. Review Common Responsibilities in Chapter 2.

b. Review Unit Leader Responsibilities in Chapter 2.

c. Review incident needs and any special procedures with Unit Leaders, as needed.

d. Coordinate with local jurisdiction on plans and supply sources.

e. Obtain the Incident Procurement Plan.

f. Prepare and authorize contracts, building and land-use agreements.

g. Draft memoranda of understanding as necessary.

h. Establish contracts and agreements with supply vendors.

i. Provide for coordination between the ORDM and all other procurement organizations supporting the incident.

j. Ensure that a system is in place that meets agency property management requirements. Ensure proper accounting for all new property.

k. Interpret contracts and agreements; resolve disputes within delegated authority.

l. Coordinate with the Compensation/Claims Unit for processing claims.

m. Complete final processing of contracts and send documents for payment.

n. Coordinate cost data in contracts with the COST.

o. Brief the FSC on current problems and recommendations, outstanding issues and follow-up requirements.

p. Maintain Unit Log (ICS 214-CG).

COMPENSATION/CLAIMS UNIT LEADER (COMP) -
The COMP is responsible for the overall management and direction of all administrative matters pertaining to compensation for injury and claims related activities (other than injury) for an incident.
The major responsibilities of the COMP are:

a. Review Common Responsibilities in Chapter 2.

b. Review Unit Leader Responsibilities in Chapter 2.

   c. Obtain a briefing from the FSC.
   d. Establish contact with the incident MEDL, SOFR
       and LNO (or Agency Representatives if no LNO
       is assigned).
   e. Determine the need for Compensation for Injury
       and Claims Specialists and order personnel as
       needed.
   f. Establish a Compensation for Injury work area
       within or as close as possible to the Medical Unit.
   g. Review Incident Medical Plan(ICS 206-CG)
   h. Ensure that CLMS's have adequate workspace
       and supplies.
   i. Review and coordinate procedures for handling
       claims with the Procurement Unit.
   j. Brief the CLMS's on incident activity.
   k. Periodically review logs and forms produced by
       the CLMS's to ensure that they are complete,
       entries are timely and accurate, and that they are
       in compliance with agency requirements and
       policies.
   l. Ensure that all Compensation for Injury and
       Claims logs and forms are complete and routed
       to the appropriate agency for post-incident
       processing prior to demobilization.
   m. Keep the FSC briefed on Unit status and activity.
   n. Demobilize unit in accordance with the Incident
       Demobilization Plan.
   o. Maintain Unit Log (ICS 214-CG).

COMPENSATION FOR INJURY SPECIALIST (INJR) -
Under the supervision of the COMP, the Compensation
for Injury Specialist is responsible for administering
financial matters resulting from serious injuries and
fatalities occurring on an incident. Close coordination is
required with the Medical Unit.
The major responsibilities of the INJR are:
   a. Review Common Responsibilities in Chapter 2.

10-7

b. Collocate Compensation for Injury Specialist with the Medical Unit when possible.
c. Establish procedure with Medical Unit Leader on prompt notification of injuries or fatalities.
d. Obtain a copy of Incident Medical Plan (ICS 206-CG).
e. Provide written authority for persons requiring medical treatment.
f. Ensure that correct agency forms are being used.
g. Provide correct billing forms for transmittal to doctor and/or hospital.
h. Coordinate with MEDL to keep informed on status of injured and/or hospitalized personnel.
i. Obtain all witness statements from SOFR and/or MEDL and review for completeness.
j. Maintain a log of all injuries occurring at the incident.
k. Coordinate/handle all administrative paperwork on serious injuries or fatalities.
l. Coordinate with appropriate agency(s) to assume responsibility for injured personnel in local hospitals after demobilization.
m. Maintain Unit Log (ICS 214-CG).

CLAIMS SPECIALIST (CLMS) - Under the supervision of the COMP, the CLMS is responsible for managing all claims-related activities (other than injury) for an incident.
The major responsibilities of the CLMS are:
a. Review Common Responsibilities in Chapter 2.
b. Develop and maintain a log of potential claims.
c. Coordinate a claims prevention plan with applicable incident functions.
d. Initiate an investigation on all claims other than personnel injury.
e. Ensure that site and property involved in an investigation are protected.

10-8

   f.   Coordinate with the investigation team as necessary.

   g.   Obtain witness statements pertaining to claims other than personnel injury.

   h.   Document any incomplete investigations.

   i.   Document follow-up action needs by the local agency.

   j.   Keep the COMP advised on the nature and status of all existing and potential claims.

   k.   Ensure the use of correct agency forms.

   l.   Maintain Unit Log (ICS 214-CG).

COST UNIT LEADER (COST) - The COST is responsible for collecting all cost data, performing cost effectiveness analyses and providing cost estimates and cost saving recommendations for the incident. The major responsibilities of the COST are:

   a.   Review Common Responsibilities in Chapter 2.

   b.   Review Unit Leader Responsibilities in Chapter 2.

   c.   Obtain a briefing from the FSC.

   d.   Coordinate with agency headquarters on cost reporting procedures.

   e.   Collect and record all cost data.

   f.   Develop incident cost summaries.

   g.   Prepare resources-use cost estimates for the Planning Section.

   h.   Make cost-saving recommendations to the FSC.

   i.   Ensure all cost documents are accurately prepared.

   j.   Maintain cumulative incident cost records.

   k.   Complete all records prior to demobilization.

   l.   Provide reports to the FSC.

   m.   Maintain Unit Log (ICS 214-CG).

TECHNICAL SPECIALISTS (THSP) – Certain incidents or events may require the use of THSP's who have specialized knowledge and expertise. THSP's may function within the Planning Section or be assigned wherever their services are required. See chapter 8 and the THSP Job Aid for more detailed information on THSP's.

FINANCE/ADMIN   **FINANCE/ADMIN**

CHAPTER 11

INTELLIGENCE

References:
- (a) National Response Plan (NRP)
- (b) National Incident Management System (NIMS)
- (c) Intelligence Officer Job Aid

INTRODUCTION

This is a brief summary of the Intelligence function as used in NIMS ICS. The Intelligence Function has been described in more detail in references (a) and (b) and a Job Aid has been developed to assist Coast Guard Intelligence Officers (reference (c)). The analysis and sharing of information and intelligence are important elements of ICS. In this context, intelligence includes not only national security or other types of classified information but also other operational information, such as risk assessments, medical intelligence (i.e., surveillance), weather information, geospatial data, structural designs, toxic contaminant levels, and utilities and public works data that may come from a variety of different sources. Traditionally, information and intelligence functions are located in the Situation Unit under the Planning Section. However, in exceptional situations, the IC/UC may need to assign the information and intelligence functions to other parts of the ICS organization. In any case, information and intelligence must be appropriately analyzed and shared with personnel, designated by the IC, who have proper clearance and a "need-to-know" to ensure that they support decision-making.

The intelligence and information function may be organized in one of the following ways:

INTELLIGENCE   **INTELLIGENCE**

a. Within the Command Staff as the <u>Intelligence Officer (INTO)</u>. This option may be most appropriate in incidents in which incident-related intelligence is provided through real-time reach-back capabilities.

b. As an <u>Intelligence Unit</u> within the Planning Section. This option may be most appropriate in an incident with some need for tactical intelligence that can be handled by the Planning Section but requires a separate unit from the Situation Unit to handle it.

c. As an <u>Intelligence Branch or Group</u> within the Operations Section. This option may be most appropriate in incidents with a high need for **tactical** intelligence actions.

d. As a separate General Staff <u>Intelligence Section</u>. This option may be most appropriate when an incident is heavily influenced by intelligence factors or when there is a need to manage and/or analyze a large volume of classified or highly sensitive intelligence or information. This option is particularly relevant to a terrorism incident, for which intelligence plays a crucial role throughout the incident life cycle.

e. As an <u>Intelligence Technical Specialist</u>. This option can be used for any situation because a technical specialist can be assigned where most needed to in the ICS organization but may be most appropriate when little intelligence information is required by the incident.

Regardless of how it is organized, the information and intelligence function is also responsible for developing, conducting, and managing information- related security plans and operations as directed by the IC. These can include information security and operational security activities, as well as the complex task of ensuring that sensitive information of all types (e.g., classified

11-2

information, sensitive law enforcement information, proprietary and personal information, or export-controlled information) is handled in a way that not only safeguards the information but also ensures that it gets to those who need access to it so that they can effectively and safely conduct their missions. The information and intelligence function also has the responsibility for coordinating information-security and operational-security matters with public awareness activities that fall under the responsibility of the PIO, particularly where such public awareness activities may affect information or operations security.

ORGANIZATION CHART
Locations where Intelligence may be located in the ICS Organization

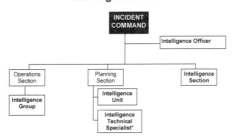

* May be assigned wherever their services are required.

For the U.S. Coast Guard, the intelligence function often fits best as the Intelligence Officer because of the Sector organization and other reasons noted in reference (c). See references (a) and (b) for more information on intelligence function and Chapter 6 and reference (c) for more information on the INTO duties and responsibilities.

THIS PAGE INTENTIONALLY LEFT BLANK

CHAPTER 12

ORGANIZATIONAL GUIDES

INCIDENT COMMAND SYSTEM
ORGANIZATION CHART

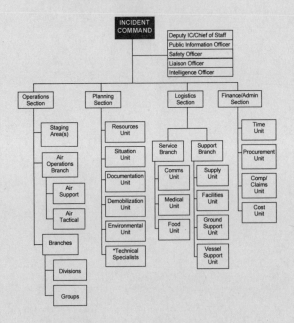

* May be assigned wherever their services are required.

ICS ORGANIZATION GUIDE

C O M M A N D

1. Incident Commander - one per incident. Unless incident is multi-jurisdictional.
2. Multi-jurisdictional incidents establish Unified Command with each jurisdiction supplying an individual to represent agency in Unified Command Structure.
3. Incident Commander may have Deputy IC's as needed.
4. Command Staff Officer - one per function per incident.
5. Command Staff may have assistants as needed.
6. Agency Representatives report to Liaison Officer on Command Staff.

INCIDENT BASE RECOMMENDED MINIMUM PERSONNEL REQUIREMENTS
(PER TWELVE (12) HOUR OPERATIONAL PERIOD or SHIFT)

(If camps are established, the minimum personnel requirements for the Base may be modified or additional personnel may be added to support camps.)

UNIT POSITION	SIZE OF INCIDENT (NUMBER OF DIVISIONS/GROUPS)				
	2	5	10	15	25
OPERATIONS					
Operations Section Chief	One Per Operational Period				
Deputy Operations Section Chief	1	1	1	2	3
Branch Director		2	3	4	6
Division/Group Supervisor	2	5	10	15	25
Strike Team Leaders	As Needed				
Task Force Leaders	As Needed				
Air Operations Director		1	1	1	1
Air Tactical Group Supervisor	1	1	1	1	1
Helicopter Coordinator	As Needed				
Air Support Group Supervisor	1	1	1	1	1
Helibase Manager	One Per Helibase				
Helispot Manager	One Per Helispot				
Staging Area Manager	One Per Staging Area				
PLANNING					
Planning Section Chief	One Per Incident				
Deputy Planning Section Chief	1	1	1	2	3
Resource Unit Leader	1	1	1	1	1
Assistant Resource Unit Leader			1	1	2
Status Recorders	1	2	3	3	4
Check-In Recorders	As Needed				
Technical Specialists	As Needed				
Situation Unit Leader	1	1	1	1	1
Assistant Situation Unit Leader			1	1	2
Display/Report Processor		1	1	1	2
SITREP/OPSUM Processors	1	1	1	2	2
Field Observer		1	2	2	4
Weather Observer	As Needed				
Aerial/Ortho Photo Analyst	As Needed				
Computer Terminal Operator		1	1	1	1
Environmental Unit Leader	1	1	1	1	1
Documentation Unit Leader		1	1	1	1
Demobilization Unit Leader			1	1	1
Demob Recorders from Resources	As Needed				

ICS Organization Guide continued

UNIT POSITION	SIZE OF INCIDENT (NUMBER OF DIVISIONS/GROUPS)				
	2	5	10	15	25
L O G I S T I C S Logistics Section Chief	One Per Incident				
Deputy Logistics Section Chief				1	2
Service Branch Director	As Needed				
Communications Unit Leader	1	1	1	1	1
Assistant Communications Unit Leader			1	1	2
Incident Communications Manager	1	1	1	1	1
Incident Dispatcher	1	2	3	3	4
Message Center Operator		1	1	2	2
Messenger		1	2	2	2
Communications Technician		1	2	4	4
Medical Unit Leader	1	1	1	1	1
Assistant Medical Unit Leader	As Needed				
Food Unit Leader		1	1	1	1
Food Unit Assistant (each camp)	As Needed				
Support Branch Director	As Needed				
Supply Unit Leader		1	1	1	1
Camp Supply Assistant (each camp)	As Needed				
Ordering Manager			1	1	1
Receiving/Distribution Manager		1	1	1	1
Recorders		1	1	2	2
Supply Unit Staff		2	2	2	2
Facility Unit Leader		1	1	1	1
Base Manager		1	1	1	1
Camp Manager (each camp)	As Needed				
Facility Maintenance Specialist		1	1	1	1
Security Manager		1	1	1	1
Facility Unit Staff		6	6	12	12
Ground Support Unit Leader	1	1	1	1	1
Equipment Manager		1	1	1	1
Assistants	As Needed				
Equipment Timekeeper		1	1	1	1
Mechanics	1	1	3	5	7
Drivers	As Needed				
Operators	As Needed				
Vessel Support Unit Leader	As Needed				
F I N - A D M I N Finance/Administration Section Chief	One Per Incident				
Deputy Finance/Admin Section Chief					1
Time Unit Leader		1	1	1	1
Time Recorder, Personnel		1	3	3	5
Time Recorder, Equipment		1	2	2	3
Procurement Unit Leader		1	1	1	1
Compensation/Claims Unit Leader		1	1	1	1
Compensation Specialist	As Needed				
Claims Specialist	As Needed				
Cost Unit Leader		1	1	1	1
Cost Analyst			1	1	1

JOINT-STAFF (J-Staff)/ICS ORGANIZATION CORRELATION CHART

Coast Guard personnel may find themselves working in a Joint-Staff (J-Staff) organization in support of DOD operations, or DOD personnel may find themselves working in support of a Federal or State Agency within an ICS organization. The following table is provided to enable those trained in an ICS position to identify where their ICS skills best fit in a J-Staff Organization. Conversely, if J-Staff qualified individuals find themselves working in an ICS organization in support of a response they can use the table to find where their J-Staff training and experience will best fit in the ICS organization.

For example, if an individual is trained as a Resources Unit Leader in ICS and they report to a J-Staff organization, their skills in ICS would best fit under J-1 (Manpower and Personnel).

* It is important to remember that the J-Staff was not intended to be an emergency response organization.

J Staff	J Staff Responsibilities	Proposed ICS Position Equivalents
Commander, Deputy Commander, Chief of Staff	◆ Plan and conduct military operations in response, including the security of the command and protection of the United States, its possessions and bases against attack or hostile incursion. ◆ Maintain the preparedness of the command to carry out missions assigned to the command. ◆ Carry out assigned missions, tasks, and responsibilities.	<u>Incident Commander</u> – the IC's responsibility is the overall management of the incident. On most incidents, a single IC carries out the command activity. The IC is selected by qualifications and experience. <u>Unified Command</u> – A unified team that manages an incident by establishing a common set of incident objectives and strategies. This is accomplished without loss or abdication of agency or organizational authority, responsibility or accountability.
Special Staff	◆ Gives technical, Administrative & tactical advice ◆ Prepares parts of plans, estimates & orders ◆ Coordinates & supervises staff active Responsible directly to the Commander	<u>Technical Specialists</u>- Personnel with special skills who can be used anywhere within the ICS Organization.
Personal Staff	◆ Gives technical, Administrative & tactical advice ◆ Prepares parts of plans, estimates & orders ◆ Coordinates & supervises staff active Responsible directly to the Commander ◆ Special Matters over which commander chooses to exercise close personal control ◆ Usually includes the political adviser ties	<u>Information Officer</u>- is responsible for developing and releasing information about the incident to the news media, to incident personnel, and to other appropriate agencies and organizations. <u>Liaison Officer</u>- is assigned to the incident to be the contact for assisting and/or cooperating Agency Representatives <u>Safety Officer</u>- to develop and recommend measures for assuring personnel safety, and to assess and/or anticipate hazardous and unsafe situations. Only the SOFR will be assigned for each incident. <u>Intelligence Officer</u>- Command Staff Officer who Determines Intelligence gaps and intelligence Requirements during the planning phase, analyzes and shares intelligence among ICS functions and involved partners, and processes classified and unclassified request for intelligence.

J Staff	J Staff Responsibilities	Proposed ICS Position Equivalents
J-1: Manpower & Personnel	♦ All matters concerning human resources and, ♦ Unit Personnel strength and readiness status ♦ Monitors and assesses elements of personnel administration & management **Receives information for coordinating, advising, and planning to assist the CG Commander in accomplishing the mission**	<u>Resources Unit</u>: Maintains status of all assigned resources at an incident (key supervisory personnel, primary & support resources, etc.). *(Planning Section)* <u>Documentation Unit</u>: Maintains accurate, up-to-date incident files. *(Planning Section)* <u>Time Unit</u>: Accurate recording of daily personnel time, compliance with time recording policies, and managing commissary operations. *(Finance/Administration Section)*
J-2: Intelligence	♦ All matters concerning military and contingency intelligence. ♦ Acquires various intelligence information and data. ♦ Analyzes and evaluates intelligence and data. ♦ Provides analyzed information and data to CG Commander with recommendations.	<u>Intel Officer</u> - Command Staff Officer who Determines Intelligence gaps and intelligence Requirements during the planning phase, analyzes and shares intelligence among ICS functions and involved partners, and processes classified and unclassified request for intelligence. The INTO manages operational information such as risk assessments, affects on public and responders, utilities and infrastructure affects, and develops strategic assessment vs. specific targeted. (Command Staff)
J-3: Operations	♦ All matters concerning contingency operations, tactical plans, tactical response organization and training ♦ Maintains current operations estimate of situation in coordination with other staff elements ♦ Coordinates & develops the operations & tactical plans, and OPORDERS ♦ Responsible for all tactical activities ♦ All personnel and unit training within Command organization	<u>Operations Section Chief</u>: Manages tactical operations, requests resources as needed, supervises execution of the Incident Action Plan for Operations, approves release of resources from assigned status. *(Operations Section)* <u>Other Branches, Task Forces, Single Resources, Staging Area Manager, Air Operations, Air Tactical Group, etc.</u> Assigned duties, as directed under the standard ICS organization. *(Operations Section)*

J Staff	J Staff Responsibilities	Proposed ICS Position Equivalents
J-4: Logistics	<ul><li>All matters concerning the response organization supplies, maintenance, transportation, and services</li><li>Determines supply requirements and coordinates/processes supply requests. Ensures supply security.</li><li>**Supervises collection, staging, distribution and transportation of supplies**</li></ul>	<u>Logistics Section Chief</u>: All incident support (exception being aviation support). *(Logistics Section)* <u>Demobilization Unit</u>: Develops Incident demobilization plan. *(Planning Section)* <u>Medical Unit</u>: Procedures for managing major medical emergencies, provide medical aid, and assist with processing injury-related claims (determine level of emergency medical activities prior to activation, acquire and manage medical support, establish procedures for handling serious injuries). *(Logistics Section)* <u>Food Unit</u>: Supplies food needs for the entire incident (determine food & water requirements, obtain necessary equipment and supplies, order sufficient food and potable water, etc.). *(Logistics Section)* <u>Supply Unit</u>: Orders, receives, processes, stores all incident-related resources. Provides supplies to planning, logistics and finance/admin sections, determines type and amount of supplies en route, orders, receives, distributes, and stores supplies and equipment, maintains inventory of supplies and equipment. *(Logistics Section)* <u>Facilities Unit</u>: Sets up, maintains and demobilizes all incident support facilities. Determines requirements for each incident facility, activates incident facilities, provides security services, etc. *(Logistics Section)* <u>Ground Support Unit</u>: Maintenance, service, and fueling of all mobile equipment & vehicles. Ground transportation of personnel, supplies and equipment. Support services for mobile equipment & vehicles, order maintenance & repair supplies, etc. *(Logistics Section)*

J Staff	J Staff Responsibilities	Proposed ICS Position Equivalents
J-4: (continued) Logistics (continued)	*(continued from previous page)*	<u>Procurement Unit</u>: All matters pertaining to vendor contracts, leases, and fiscal agreements. Coordinate with local jurisdiction on plans and supply sources, draft memoranda of understanding, establish contracts & agreements with supply vendors. *(Finance/Administration Section)*
J-5: Plans & Policy	♦ All matters concerning the long range response organization planning. ♦ Prepares mission, concept, and overall operations plans for the contingency. ♦ Prepares the recommended Course of Action (COA) and Commander's Estimates (CE), and provides response recommendations. ♦ Coordinates and facilitates all planning functions and processes.	<u>Planning Section Chief</u>: Evaluates, processes, and disseminates information for use at the incident. Reassigns out-of-service personnel already on-site to ICS organizational positions, as appropriate, establishes information requirements, and reporting schedules, determines need for any specialized resources, assembles information on alternative strategies, provides periodic predictions on incident potential, reports any significant changes in incident status. *(Planning Section)*
J-6: Command, Control & Communications	♦ All matters concerning Command, Control, and Communications. ♦ Handles command responsibilities for communications. ♦ Coordinates tactical communications planning and execution. ♦ Manages and develops the electronics and automatic information systems.	<u>Communications Unit</u>: Develops plans for the use of incident communications equipment and facilities, installs and tests the communications equipment, supervises the Incident Communications Center, distributes and maintains communications equipment. *(Communications Section)*

J-7 **Operational Plans and Interoperability**	• Prepares appropriate strategic and theater force structure recommendations and alternatives for use in the development of military plans. • Prepares the appropriate JSPS documents to support implementation of Joint Staff force structure recommendations including force apportionment and assignment. • Conducts tradeoff analyses between force effectiveness and alternative resource distributions. • Conducts tradeoff analyses of joint force capabilities and requires, including assessments of the projected readiness, sustainability, modernization, and force structure aspects of current and programmed forces.	**Planning Section Chief:** Evaluates, processes, and disseminates information for use at the incident. Reassigns out-of-service personnel already on-site to ICS organizational positions, as appropriate, establishes information requirements, and reporting schedules, determines need for any specialized resources, assembles information on alternative strategies, provides periodic predictions on incident potential, reports any significant changes in incident status. *(Planning Section)*

J-8 Force Structure, Resources and Assessment	◆ Pursues joint force development through joint doctrine, training, war plans, and assessments ◆ Through the Joint Training System, joint exercise program, CJCS Assessment Program, and review of conventional war plans, assists the combatant commands, Joint Staff, Services, and OSD to exercise and improve the capability of US forces and combat support agencies to achieve strategic goals. ◆ Facilitates addressing warfighting requirements needed in war plans, joint education, training, and doctrine.	**Finance Section Chief**- is responsible for all financial, administrative, and cost analysis aspects of the incident and for supervising members of the Finance/Administration Section. ◆ **Compensation/Claims**: Oversees completion of all forms required by workers' compensation and local agencies. Also maintains file of injuries and illnesses, associated with the incident. Close coordination with the Medical Unit. Claims are responsible for investigating all claims involving property associated with or involved in incident. *(Finance/Administration Section)* ◆ **Cost Unit**: Provides all incident cost analysis. Insures proper identification of all equipment and personnel requiring payment, prepares estimates of incident costs, and maintains accurate records of incident costs. *(Finance/Administration Section)* ◆ **Procurement Unit**: All matters pertaining to vendor contracts, leases, and fiscal agreements. Coordinate with local jurisdiction on plans and supply sources, draft memoranda of understanding, establish contracts 7 agreements with supply vendors. *(Finance/Administration Section*

JOPES and ICS Interaction

Anyone who has participated in the Joint Operational Planning and Execution System (JOPES) or ICS planning processes will understand the value of *Process*. Process is as important as and sometimes more important than the plan. The process itself drives critical information and communication of that information where it needs to go. JOPES consists of two planning processes; Crisis Action Planning (CAP) and Deliberate Planning. ICS delineates between *Unplanned Incidents* and *Planned Events*. Although ICS has been utilized for large scale Planned Events, by design, it is a CAP process.

The JOPES and ICS Interaction diagram takes the *linear* process for producing JOPES OPLANS and Orders and *bends* it around the ICS Operational Planning "P". This works because the basic functional activities are essentially the same for all planning processes. The diagram translates between JOPES and ICS functions, phases, and tools. Both JOPES and ICS practitioners can now see that the processes flow in the same sequence; how by implication, portions of a JOPES plan or order relate to ICS tools; and that continuous improvement of ICS can be incorporated into JOPES OPLANS and Orders.

Current Coast Guard doctrine dictates JOPES for some of its Deliberate Planning and ICS for most CAP responses. The Deliberate OPLANS and Contingency Plans prepare units for response and directly feed into the development of ICS Incident Action Plans when they do.

JOPES and ICS Interaction

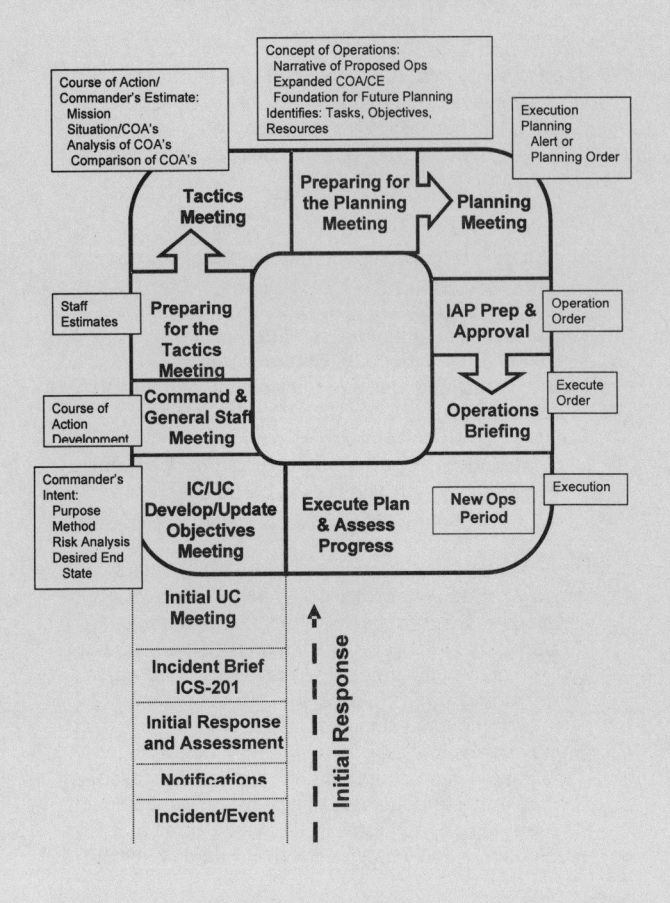

Course of Action/
Commander's Estimate:
 Mission
 Situation/COA's
 Analysis of COA's
 Comparison of COA's

Concept of Operations:
 Narrative of Proposed Ops
 Expanded COA/CE
 Foundation for Future Planning
Identifies: Tasks, Objectives,
Resources

Execution
Planning
Alert or
Planning Order

**Tactics
Meeting**

**Preparing for
the Planning
Meeting**

**Planning
Meeting**

Staff
Estimates

**Preparing
for the
Tactics
Meeting**

**IAP Prep &
Approval**

Operation
Order

Course of
Action
Development

**Command &
General Staff
Meeting**

**Operations
Briefing**

Execute
Order

Commander's
Intent:
 Purpose
 Method
 Risk Analysis
 Desired End
 State

**IC/UC
Develop/Update
Objectives
Meeting**

**Execute Plan
& Assess
Progress**

**New Ops
Period**

Execution

**Initial UC
Meeting**

**Incident Brief
ICS-201**

**Initial Response
and Assessment**

Notifications

Incident/Event

Initial Response

12-12

CHAPTER 13

AREA COMMAND

CHAPTER 13

AREA COMMAND

References:
  (a) National Response Plan (NRP)
  (b) National Incident Management System NIMS)
  (c) Area Command Job Aid
  (d) Logistics Section Chief Job Aid

INTRODUCTION

The purpose of an Area Command (AC) is to oversee the management of the incident(s), focusing primarily on strategic assistance and direction and resolving competition for scarce response resources. An Area Command (AC) is activated only if necessary, depending on the complexity of the incident and incident management span-of-control considerations. This organization does not supplant the Incident Commanders (IC's) and Unified Commands (UC's), but supports and provides strategic direction. Execution of tactical operations and coordination remains the responsibility of the on-scene incident command/unified command structure.

Area Command is an organization activated by the Sector, District, or Area Commander to ensure coordination for Command, Planning, Logistical and Fiscal matters. For example, the need for an AC may arise when there are multiple incidents and/or a spill of national significance (SONS). The AC will determine critical resource allocation. For multiple incidents, AC may also establish incident prioritization.

NOTE: For further details on operating procedures refer to the Area Command Job Aid.

AREA COMMAND
CONCEPT OF OPERATIONS

AC Activation Criteria

A District/Area Commander or the Commandant can determine when an incident(s) is of such magnitude, complexity or operational intensity that it would benefit from the activation of an AC. Also, there may be times when multiple incidents occur within one Sector Commander zone where incidents are competing for the same resources. The AC may be designated by the Sector Commander or the Sector Commander may fulfill the AC role. Factors to consider when deciding to activate an AC include but are not limited to:

1. Complex incident overwhelming local and regional Coast Guard assets;
2. An incident that overlaps Coast Guard districts;
3. An incident that crosses international borders;
4. The existence of, or the potential for, a high level of national political and media interest;
5. Significant threat or impact to the public health and welfare, natural environment, property or economy over a broad geographic area; or
6. More than one active incident where incidents are competing for the same resources.

AC Activation Guidance

When the decision is made to activate an AC, the following actions should occur:

1. An Area Commander is designated by the Sector Commander, District Commander, Area Commander or the Commandant.
2. Designated Area Commander and deputy/deputies will be delegated clear succession of command authority.
3. If an incident(s) is multi-jurisdictional, the AC shall be established using Unified Command (UC)

13-3

concepts and principles. When Unified Area Command (UAC) is established, representatives will typically consist of executives possessing the highest level of response authority as possible.
4. Determine appropriate location for the Area Command Post (ACP).

AC Responsibilities
AC has the overall responsibility for strategic management of the incident(s) and will:
1. Establish AC strategic objectives.
2. Establish overall response priorities.
3. Rank incidents in order of priority.
4. Identify and allocate critical resources based on incident needs.
5. Ensure that the incident(s) is properly managed;
6. Ensure that the on-scene incident(s) objectives are met.
7. Minimize conflict with supporting agency's/ stakeholder and public concerns.
8. Coordinate acquisition of critical or specialized resources.
9. In the event that a Joint field Office (JFO) is activated, coordinate acquisition of national assets to support the incident(s) between AC and the JFO. (See reference (a) or Chapter 14 for detailed description of a JFO.)

AC Staffing
The AC organization should be kept as small as possible. The size of the AC organization will be determined by the authorities and support requirements of the incident(s) and follows standard ICS principles like flexibility and scalability. Under normal circumstances, AC staffing will consist of:
1. Area Commander(s) and Deputy/Deputies
2. AC Liaison Officer (AC LNO)

13-4

3. AC Safety Officer (AC SOFR)
4. AC Public Information Officer (AC PIO)
5. AC Intelligence Officer (AC INTO)
6. AC Logistics Chief (AC LC)
7. AC Communication Unit Leader (AC COML)
8. AC Information Technology Specialist (AC ITS)
9. AC Facility Unit Leader (AC FACL)
10. AC Planning Chief (AC PC)
11. AC Documentation Unit Leader (AC DOCL)
12. AC Critical Resources Unit Leader (AC CRESL)
13. AC Situation Unit Leader (AC SITL)
14. AC Finance/Administration Chief (AC FC)

Optional Staffing
1. Legal Specialist
2. Security Specialist
3. Intel Specialist
4. Aviation Coordinator
5. Documentation Specialist/Executive Assistant
6. Legislative Affairs Officer

<u>**The Area Command organization does not, in any way, replace the on-scene incident organization(s) or functions.**</u> The above positions, if established, are strictly related to supporting the AC functional responsibilities. Tactical operations continue to be directed at the on-scene IC/UC command level.

In addition, **Expanded Ordering** may be set up outside of the local incident(s) and outside of Area Command to assist with non-critical resource ordering. See more about expanded ordering process in reference (d), the Logistics Section Chief Job Aid.

AC REPORTING RELATIONSHIPS

It is envisioned that the role of Area Commander for Incidents of National Significance (INS) will be filled by a Flag Officer (or their designee) with the ability to set priorities and objectives on behalf of the entire Coast Guard. When established, the Area Commander reports through normal Coast Guard reporting channels to the Commandant. If a JFO or other Multiagency Coordination Centers (MACS) are established, the AC will need to determine the appropriate level of coordination and liaison required to support the incident(s).

AREA COMMAND ORGANIZATION

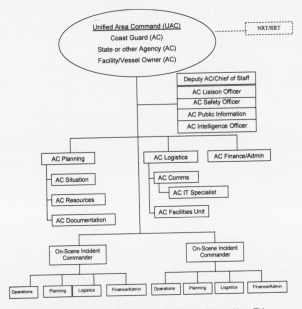

Note: NIIMS Area Command includes an Aviation Coordinator position. This position was intentionally left out for Coast Guard AC. The AC can add the position anytime they determine a need for special aviation coordination.

AREA COMMAND
POSITION CHECKLISTS

AREA COMMANDER (AC)

The Area Commander is responsible for providing the overall direction to the on-scene IC(s). This responsibility includes ensuring that conflicts are resolved, incident objectives are established and strategies are selected to meet AC priorities and strategic objectives.

The Area Commander responsibilities are as follows:
1. Review Common Responsibilities in Chapter 2.
2. Obtain authorities and policy guidance from agency executive(s).
3. Provide briefings to the next level of command through normal reporting channels.
4. If operating within a UAC, develop a working agreement with all UAC participants to ensure that jurisdictional authorities are not compromised or neglected.
5. In coordination with on-scene IC's/UC's determine level of effort AC will need to support.
6. Based on the scope of the job, ensure the AC organization is capable of meeting their functional responsibility.
7. Identify location and establish an appropriate Area Command Post.
8. Establish authorities and policy guidance and communicate to AC team members.
9. Develop overall direction, priorities, and strategic objectives and convey to on-scene IC's/UC's.
10. Ensure that the incident response strategies address the direction set by the AC.
11. Establish priorities for assignment and demobilization of critical resources.
12. Coordinate demobilization of critical resources.

13-8

13. Establish a media strategy (plan) for release of information to the media, the public, etc.
14. Serve as public spokesperson for the overall response.
15. Manage the AC organization to ensure the on-scene IC's/UC's are appropriately supported.
16. Maintain AC log of strategic decisions.
17. Monitor and evaluate AC Incident management Team (AC IMT) performance.
18. Anticipate and analyze long term big picture potential consequences and develop strategic response alternatives.

DEPUTY AREA COMMANDER (DAC)

The AC may have Deputy AC's, who may be from the same agency or from an assisting agency. The Deputy AC must have the same qualifications as the person for whom they work, as they must be ready to take over that position at any time. When span of control becomes an issue for the AC, a Deputy AC/Chief of Staff may be assigned to manage the AC Command Staff.

The major responsibilities of the DAC are:

1. Review Common Responsibilities in Chapter 2.
2. Assist the AC in executing their responsibilities.
3. Perform Area Commander Duties in the absence of the designated Area Commander.
4. Oversee and facilitate the overall operation of the AC Staff and General Staff functions on behalf of the Area Commander.
5. Administer special projects as assigned.

AC LIAISON OFFICER (AC LNO)

Establish liaison, as needed, with representatives of assisting and cooperating agencies. This will often be with the same agencies represented at the IC level, but will typically be a link to a more senior organizational level than that represented on-scene.

The major responsibilities of the AC LNO are:

1. Review Common Responsibilities in Chapter 2.
2. Review the LNO Job Aid.
3. Establish liaison, as needed, with stakeholders, such as environmental, economic, and political groups. It is expected, however, that the majority of stakeholder service and support will be handled at the on-scene command level.
4. Support on-scene LNO(s) efforts to establish strong ties with assisting/cooperating agencies and stakeholders.
5. When appropriate coordinate with the National Response Team (NRT)/Regional Response Team (RRT) to identify and resolve issues and concerns.
6. Maintain communications with stakeholders and assisting and cooperating agencies and keep AC advised of their issues and concerns.
7. Liaise with all investigating agencies, to minimize impact on incident response operations.
8. Coordinate AC site visits with on-scene command.

AC PUBLIC INFORMATION OFFICER (AC PIO)

The AC PIO is responsible for developing and releasing information about the incident to the news media, to incident personnel, and to other appropriate agencies and organizations. Normally, detailed information regarding response specifics will be referred to and handled by the appropriate on-scene PIO. The AC PIO will generally provide information on overall progress and status of the response from a regional or national perspective.

The major responsibilities of the AC PIO are:

1. Review Common Responsibilities in Chapter 2.
2. Review the PIO and JIC Job Aids.

3. Provide information on the incident(s) to the media and other interested parties.
4. Identify and communicate to AC organization and on-scene IMT, the Area Command's policy and procedures for release of information.
5. As directed, establish and manage the AC Joint Information Center (AC JIC).
6. Coordinate with the on-scene PIO(s) to obtain information and to ensure consistency in release of information.
7. Closely coordinate with on-scene PIO's to develop and establish an effective public information strategy.
8. Evaluate public and media perception of the response effectiveness and keep AC and on-scene command informed.
9. Keep the AC and AC staff informed of news releases, press conferences, town meetings, etc., to be conducted at the AC level.
10. Prepare briefing materials and coordinate the conduct of press conferences, town meetings, etc.
11. Provide speaker preparation and coaching to members of the AC staff.
12. Carry out the protocol function for visiting dignitaries, including coordination and conduct of briefs and site visits. As much as possible, AC will coordinate VIP site visits in an effort to minimize the impact on the on-scene IMT's.

AC SAFETY OFFICER (AC SOFR)

The SOFR function is to develop and recommend measures for assuring personnel safety and to assess and/or anticipate hazardous and unsafe situations. Normally, detailed information regarding response specifics will be referred to and handled by the appropriate on-scene SOFR. The AC SOFR will generally provide information on overall safety issues

13-11

and progress/status of the response from a regional or
national perspective.
The major responsibilities of the AC SOFR are:
1. Review Common Responsibilities in Chapter 2.
2. Review the SOFR Job Aid.
3. Develop AC Facility Safety Plan and monitor for
   compliance.
4. Evaluate thoroughness of the on-scene Site Safety
   Plan(s).
5. As requested, provide assistance to on-scene
   SOFR and on-scene IMT's in investigating
   accidents, injuries, fatalities, etc.
6. Review on-scene Incident Action Plans (IAP's) for
   safety implications.

AC INTELLIGENCE OFFICER (AC INTO)

For the U.S. Coast Guard, the intelligence function has
been determined to best fit as the INTO. For more
information on the Intelligence function, see Chapter
11. The responsibility of the AC INTO is to provide
Command intelligence information for the AC that can
have a direct impact on the response personnel and
influence the disposition of maritime security assets
involved in the response. Normally, detailed information
regarding incident intelligence specifics will be referred
to and handled by the appropriate on-scene INTO. The
AC INTO will generally provide information on overall
intelligence issues and progress/status of the response
from a regional or national perspective.
The major responsibilities of the AC INTO are:
1. Review Common Responsibilities in Chapter 2.
2. Review the INTO Job Aid.
3. Working with AC, determine the level and
   complexity of Intelligence needed to support their
   efforts.

13-12

4. Reach agreement with AC on where the intelligence position will be located within the AC organization.
5. Determine Intelligence gaps and Intelligence requirements needed to support AC's decision making process and the development of the Operating Guide.
6. Analyze and share intelligence among AC organization, involved partners and the on-scene IMT(s).
7. Manage and process classified and unclassified requests for intelligence.
8. Ensure that intelligence is properly used and filed.
9. Coordinate intelligence gathering activities with other external agencies and organizations (i.e. FBI, State and local law enforcement, etc).

AC PLANNING CHIEF (AC PC)

The AC Planning Chief is responsible for collecting, evaluating, managing, and disseminating information at the AC level. The responsibility of the AC PC is to provide AC planning information for the AC that can have a direct impact on the response personnel and influence the disposition of maritime security assets involved in the response. Normally, detailed information regarding incident planning specifics will be referred to and handled by the appropriate on-scene PSC. The AC PC will generally provide information on overall planning issues and progress/status of the response from a regional or national perspective.

The major responsibilities of the AC PC are:
1. Review Common Responsibilities in Chapter 2.
2. Review the PSC Job Aid.
3. Review on-scene incident action plans for purposes of assessing potential conflicts with AC direction.
4. Oversee the preparation and dissemination of the AC Operating Guide (OG).

5. Facilitate/conduct AC meetings and briefings.
6. Prepare material and conduct special situation briefings for AC.
7. Assure appropriate displays are developed, maintained and posted.
8. Ensure all off-site reporting requirements are met, i.e., ICS 209-CG.
9. Ensure a documentation process is in place for collecting, duplicating and filing information, including intelligence.
10. Brief Operating Guide to AC staff, Agency Executives, on-scene commanders and VIP's.
11. Ensure that the on-scene commander(s) are adequately anticipating and developing contingencies for addressing future response needs.
12. Assist AC in the development of strategies, objectives, priorities, operating procedures and protocols.
13. Coordinate with Logistics on the identification of, ordering, assignment and demobilization of critical resources.
14. Ensure accurate status of critical resources.
15. Prepare and distribute the AC policies, procedures and decisions to the AC staff and the on-scene IC's/UC's.
16. Ensure a check-in process is in place to ensure accountability of visitors and command post personnel.
17. Develop recommendation for standing down the AC organization (demobilization).

AC SITUATION UNIT LEADER (AC SITL)

The AC SITL is responsible for collecting, processing and organizing incident information relating to the growth, mitigation or intelligence activities taking place on the incident. The SITL may prepare future projections of incident growth, maps and intelligence information. The responsibility of the AC SITL is to provide situational information for the AC that can have a direct impact on the response personnel and influence the disposition of maritime security assets involved in the response. The AC SITL will generally provide information on overall issues and progress/status of the response from a regional or national perspective.

The major responsibilities of the AC PC are:

1. Review Common Responsibilities in Chapter 2.
2. Review the SITL Job Aid.
3. Develop and implement procedures for collecting and displaying the current operational picture that reflects AC overall response emphasis.
4. Collect and analyze intelligence gathered from on-scene command, external entities, AC staff, and brief AC on the potential implications.
5. Maintain current situation status displays.
6. Prepare incident situation information for support of, and use in, meetings, briefings and reporting documents.
7. Prepare for and conduct situation briefings.
8. Establish and maintain a task/action tracking process (ICS-234-CG).
9. Develop and maintain ICS 209AC-CG, Incident Status Summary.
10. As scheduled, provide frequent/timely incident status updates (ICS 209AC-CG) to Coast Guard Headquarters, the parent Coast Guard District, and other agencies and entities.
11. Be prepared to respond to real-time critical information requests.
12. As required, provide incident status updates to stakeholders or other external organizations on an unscheduled basis.

13-15

13. Develop and post a briefing and meeting schedule ICS 230AC-CG.
14. Develop a list of critical information elements.

AC CRITICAL RESOURCES UNIT LEADER (AC CRESL)

The AC CRESL is responsible for maintaining the status of all critical tactical resources and personnel. The AC CRESL will generally provide information on critical resources issues and progress/status of the response from a regional or national perspective.

The major responsibilities of the AC CRESL are:

1. Review Common Responsibilities in Chapter 2.
2. Review RESL Job Aid.
3. Maintain resource status for all critical resources.
4. Maintain resource status on all AC organization.
5. Establish and maintain a check-in process to ensure accountability of visitors and command post personnel.
6. Develop and post an AC organization chart ICS AC207-CG.
7. Assist Planning Chief in the development and assembling of the AC Operating Guide.
8. Support/assist the AC Planning Chief in assigning and demobilizing critical resources.
9. Develop 24 hr watch schedule.
10. Working with the on-scene commanders, submit critical resource needs to the AC Logistics Chief.
11. Coordinate with the AC Finance/Administration Chief to track response costs for AC.
12. Develop and maintain the Resource Allocation and Prioritization worksheet ICS AC215-CG.
13. Set-up meeting and briefing area using the meeting room layout (Refer to Area Command job aid for room layout).

AC DOCUMENTATION UNIT LEADER (AC DOCL)

The DOCL is responsible for the maintenance of accurate, up-to-date incident files.

The major responsibilities of the AC DOCL are:

1. Review Common Responsibilities in Chapter 2.
2. Review the DOCL Job Aid.
3. Establish a process for collecting, analyzing and storing AC documentation both non-secure and secure information.
4. Establish duplication service and respond to requests.
5. File all official memos, forms and reports.
6. Enforce confidentiality policies on release of documents.
7. Monitor accuracy of completeness of records submitted for filing.
8. Provide duplicates of forms and reports to authorized requesters.
9. Obtain approval for release of any documents or reports.
10. Prepare final files for hand-off to appropriate official for future use.

AC LOGISTICS CHIEF (AC LC)

The responsibility of the AC LC is responsible to provide facilities, services, and material in support of the AC.

The major responsibilities of the AC LC are:

1. Review Common Responsibilities in Chapter 2.
2. Review the LSC Job Aid.
3. Establish and maintain an appropriate ACP for the AC organization.
4. Provide services, and support for the AC organization, including billeting, transportation, feeding, etc.
5. Respond to requests to meet AC organization staffing requirements.

13-17

6. Establish and maintain a resource ordering process for the AC organization.
7. Work with on-scene IMT's to identify and respond to critical resource needs.
8. Identify list of potential critical/specialized resource suppliers.
9. Source, order and track critical and specialized resources from point of departure to incident check-in.
10. Support/assist the Planning Chief, in developing recommendations for establishing priorities to govern the assignment and demobilization of critical resources.
11. Plan for, and establish secure and non-secure voice and data communication for internal and external needs of the AC organization.
12. As appropriate, provide security services for the ACP.
13. When directed by AC, take charge of the expanded supply network to support the on-scene commanders.
14. Develop AC Communication Plan, ICS AC205-CG.
15. Establish and maintain an accountable-property tracking system.
16. Coordinate directly with the Finance/Administration Chief, for procurement and accounting purposes.

AC FACILITIES UNIT LEADER (AC FACL)
The AC FACL is primarily responsible for the set up, maintenance and demobilization of AC facilities.
The major responsibilities of the AC FACL are:
1. Review Common Responsibilities in Chapter 2.
2. Determine space requirements for ACP.
3. Prepare ACP footprint and assist AC staff in setting up individual work areas.
4. Coordinate with Safety Officer in conducting Site Safety Inspection of ACP.

5. If required, provide for billeting and feeding of AC personnel.
6. Provide for facility maintenance (e.g. sanitation, janitorial services, lighting, etc.).
7. Ensure facility is maintained in a safe condition.
8. Restore facility to its pre-occupancy condition.
9. If required, develop Facility Security Plan and manage security activities including staff parking area.
10. Ensure that all facility equipment is acquired, setup and properly functioning (i.e. furniture, display boards, copy machines, faxes, etc).
11. Establish property accountability system for issued equipment.

AC COMMUNICATIONS UNIT LEADER (AC COML)

The AC COML is responsible for developing plans for the effective use of AC communications equipment and facilities; installing and testing of communications equipment; supervision of the AC Communications Center.

The major responsibilities of the AC COML are:
1. Review Common Responsibilities in Chapter 2.
2. Review COML Job Aid.
3. Prepare and implement AC Communications Plan for both internal and external needs.
4. Provide input into the AC Operating guide as it relates to communications, ICS AC205-CG.
5. Ensure communications systems are installed and tested and maintained including ACP internal telephone system.
6. Coordinate with on-scene communication Unit Leaders and assist with acquisition of specialized equipment and frequency management issues.
7. Provide technical information to both the ACP staff and incident(s).

8. Establish accountability system for issued communications equipment.
9. If required, install secure communication network.

AC INFORMATION TECHNOLOGY SPECIALIST (AC ITS)

The major responsibilities of the AC ITS are:
1. Review Common Responsibilities in Chapter 2.
2. Analyze the requirements for data processing to support the ACP for both internal and external data transmission needs (for both secure and non-secure).
3. Install and maintain ACP LAN and stand alone system including laptops, printers and plotters.
4. Brief user group on system operations.
5. Based on requirements, determine need for specialized expertise to operate and maintain systems.

AC FINANCE CHIEF (AC FC)

The AC FC is responsible for all financial, administrative and cost analysis aspects of the AC and for supervising members of the AC Finance/Admin Section.

The major responsibilities of the AC FC are:
1. Review Common Responsibilities in Chapter 2.
2. Review the FSC Job Aid.
3. Determine Area Command requirements for cost accounting.
4. Coordinate with on-scene Finance/Admin Section Chief(s) to determine methodology for reporting cost information.
5. Collect, analyze and summarize cost data.
6. Keep AC briefed on response costs.
7. Ensure that response costs are managed within the established financial ceilings and guidelines.

13-20

8. Coordinate and advise AC on ceiling adjustments when necessary.
9. For oil and hazardous materials incidents: keep the AC advised as to the impact on the Oil Spill Liability Trust Fund (OSLTF) or CERCLA Fund and potential/projected time for reaching liability limits of the Facility/Vessel owner .
10. Establish a Pollution Removal Funding Authorization (PRFA) or other interagency agreements and ensure compliance with all cost documentation requirements of interagency fiscal agreements.
11. For oil spills: Coordinate the overall processing of claims with the Facility/Vessel owner and on-scene Finance/Admin Section Chiefs.
12. Coordinate with JFO for Stafford Act funding sources.
13. If required, develop cost sharing agreements with member of AC.
14. Monitor use of high cost specialized equipment and keep AC advised.
15. If required, coordinate processing of claims resulting from response actions.

OPTIONAL POSITIONS/TECHNICAL SPECIALISTS

LAW SPECIALIST
1. Review Common Responsibilities in Chapter 2.
2. Review Technical Specialist Job Aid.
3. Advise the AC on legal issues.
4. Establish links with the Facility/Vessel owner, state, and other applicable legal representatives. This is primarily a responsibility during Spills of National Significance (SONS).
5. Review documents developed by AC or AC staff to ensure they meet the legal requirements of participating agencies and organizations.

6. Ensure AC documentation control system is appropriate.
7. Identify what documents and/or information can or cannot be released during the response.
8. Monitor compliance of agreements being used during the response (i.e. MEXUS, etc.).

SECURITY SPECIALIST

1. Review Common Responsibilities in Chapter 2.
2. Review Technical Specialist Job Aid.
3. Determine security requirements of the Area Command Post (ACP).
4. Develop and implement ACP Security Plan.
5. Obtain assets to monitor and enforce security.
6. If required, determine need for ACP identification badge system and provide this service.
7. Evaluate and recommend to AC the need for secure communications for both voice and data.
8. Coordinate with on-scene security specialist(s) as needed to ensure security requirements are met.
9. If needed, establish a list of ACP personnel levels of security clearance.

AVIATION COORDINATOR

1. Review Common Responsibilities in Chapter 2.
2. Determine where in the AC organization this function will be assigned.
3. Determine AC requirements for use of aviation assets.
4. If aviation assets are determined to be a critical resource, coordinate with the Planning and Logistics Chief on ordering, assigning and demobilizing these assets.
5. Schedule the use of aviation assets assigned to support AC and their staff.
6. Coordinate with the On-scene Air Operations Director for multi- incident utilization of air assets.

13-22

7. Provide technical expertise on the use of specialized air assets to both AC and on-scene IMT(s).
8. If needed, develop an ICS 220-CG, Air Operations Summary Work Sheet.

DOCUMENTATION SPECIALIST/EXECUTIVE ASSISTANT

1. Review Common Responsibilities in Chapter 2.
2. Review Technical Specialist and DOCL Job Aids.
3. Determine AC requirements for documenting meeting and briefing.
4. Prepare Decision Memos for AC and primary staff review and approval.
5. Ensure AC meeting notes accurately reflect what was said.
6. Ensure that AC meeting notes, memos and reports are provided to the Documentation Unit Leader.
7. Develop and maintain chronological Log of AC decisions, direction and actions.
8. Perform other administractive duties as may be assigned (i.e. runner, expeditor, etc.).

AREA COMMAND OPERATING CYCLE MEETINGS, BRIEFINGS, AND THE OPERATING GUIDE PROCESS

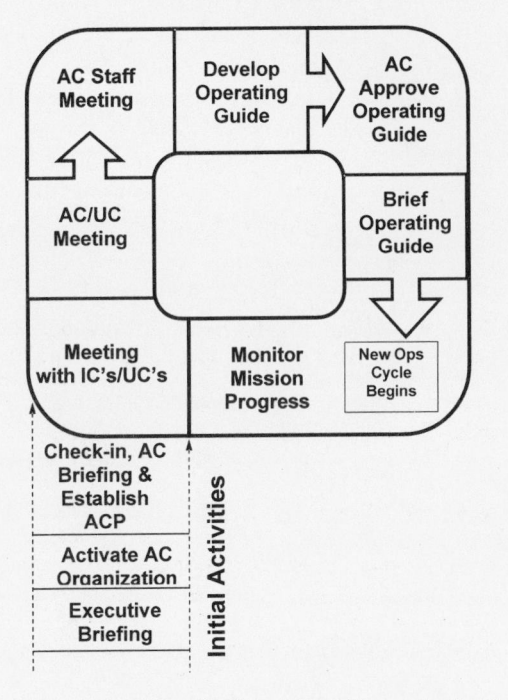

The period of initial activation of the AC organization is when a determination is made to establish an AC organization to support on-scene IMT's. Senior Agency Representatives/Agency Executive(s) determine and designate who will represent the Coast Guard and other appropriate organizations within the AC structure.

13-24

EXECUTIVE BRIEFING – This is the first activity where the representatives in Area Command are briefed by senior agency executives on the overall situation which includes:

- Establish authorities.
- Receive policy guidance.
- Reach agreement on the scope of the job.
- Identify Area Command Post location.

When: Selected Area Commander(s) gather for the first time

Facilitator: Senior Agency Executive or designee

Attendees: Selected Area Commanders and deputies

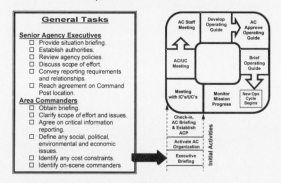

General Tasks

Senior Agency Executives
☐ Provide situation briefing.
☐ Establish authorities.
☐ Review agency policies.
☐ Discuss scope of effort.
☐ Convey reporting requirements and relationships.
☐ Reach agreement on Command Post location.

Area Commanders
☐ Obtain briefing.
☐ Clarify scope of effort and issues.
☐ Agree on critical information reporting.
☐ Define any social, political, environmental and economic issues.
☐ Identify any cost constraints.
☐ Identify on-scene commanders

EXECUTIVE BRIEFING AGENDA

1. Brief on the need and requirements for AC organization.
2. Discuss prior communications between executives and IC's/UC's.
3. Brief on current situation.
4. Brief on AC authorities, duties and responsibilities.

13-25

5. Discuss overarching political, social, economic and environmental issues affecting the mission.
6. Clarify reporting and briefing requirements and lines of authority.
7. Discuss and reach agreement on overall AC staffing and Area Command Post (ACP) location.
8. Discuss plans and agreements that may be in place.
9. Close out meeting with concurrence from Area Commanders that their concerns have been addressed.

ACTIVATE AC ORGANIZATION/INITIAL AC MEETING – Provides Area Commander(s) the opportunity to determine the size of the Area Command organization based on the scope of effort and agreements reached at the Executive Briefing. This time block could also be used to evaluate the suitability of the proposed ACP location to meet AC organizational needs. Area Commander(s) come to agreement on AC staffing.

When: Shortly after the Executive Briefing
Facilitator: AC Member or AC PC (if available)
Attendees: Area Commanders

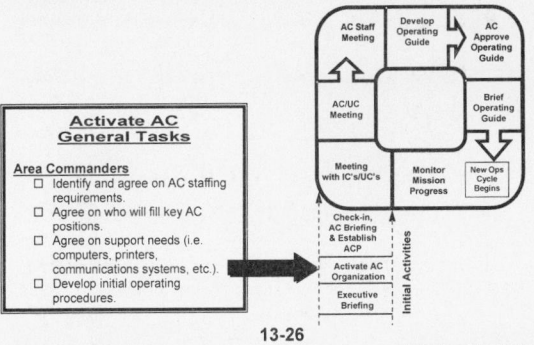

Activate AC
General Tasks

Area Commanders
☐ Identify and agree on AC staffing requirements.
☐ Agree on who will fill key AC positions.
☐ Agree on support needs (i.e. computers, printers, communications systems, etc.).
☐ Develop initial operating procedures.

13-26

ACTIVATE AC ORGANIZATION/INITIAL AC MEETING AGENDA:

1. Facilitator brings meeting to order, covers ground rules and reviews agenda.
2. Validate makeup of newly formed UAC, based on Chapter 5 criteria.
3. Clarify UAC Roles and Responsibilities.
4. Review agency policies.
5. Establish and document response Priorities, Limitations and Constraints.
6. Define and document the UAC jurisdictional boundaries and focus (Area of Responsibility (AOR)).
7. Determine location of Area Command Post (ACP).
8. Determine AC period length/start time and work shift hours.
9. Designate lead organization for AC Planning Chief, Information, Safety, Intelligence and Liaison Officers as needed.
10. Designate other AC key staff assignments as needed.
11. Discuss and agree on managing sensitive information, resource ordering, cost sharing, cost accounting, and operational security issues.
12. Summarize and document key decisions, procedures and guidance.

CHECK-IN, AC STAFF BRIEFING & ESTABLISH ACP

– Area Commanders will conduct initial briefing with AC personnel. Briefing will include expectations from Area Commanders and any limitations or issues the AC will be expected to address. Establishment of the ACP may also be addressed at this time.

When: At the time AC staff begins to arrive and ACP is being established

Facilitator: AC PC or Area Commander(s) with participation from Planning and Logistics Chiefs

Attendees: All AC personnel

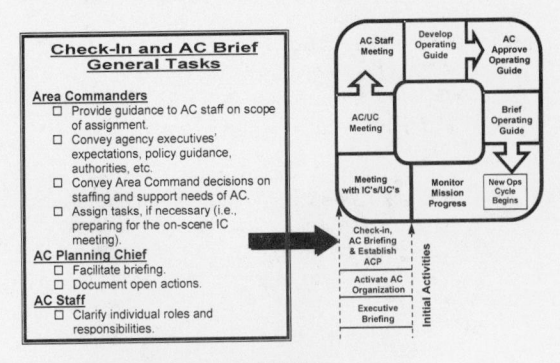

Check-In and AC Brief General Tasks

Area Commanders
☐ Provide guidance to AC staff on scope of assignment.
☐ Convey agency executives' expectations, policy guidance, authorities, etc.
☐ Convey Area Command decisions on staffing and support needs of AC.
☐ Assign tasks, if necessary (i.e., preparing for the on-scene IC meeting).

AC Planning Chief
☐ Facilitate briefing.
☐ Document open actions.

AC Staff
☐ Clarify individual roles and responsibilities.

AC STAFF MEETING AGENDA:

1. AC PC brings meeting to order, conducts roll call, covers ground rules and reviews agenda.
2. AC SITL conducts situation status briefing.
3. AC provides initial comments, expectations, initial assignments, and closing comments.

MEETING WITH ON-SCENE INCIDENT COMMANDERS/UNIFIED COMMANDS – Provides

Area Commander(s) the opportunity to dialogue with on-scene IC's/UC's and receive on-scene IC's/UC's current situation, strategies and issues confronting them.

When: As soon as possible after AC becomes operational

Facilitator: AC PC

Attendees: Area Commanders, Planning, Logistics and Finance/Admin Chiefs, On-scene IC's/UC's and their Planning Section Chiefs

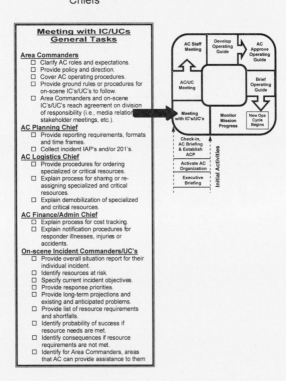

Meeting with IC/UCs General Tasks

Area Commanders
- ☐ Clarify AC roles and expectations.
- ☐ Provide policy and direction.
- ☐ Cover AC operating procedures.
- ☐ Provide ground rules or procedures for on-scene IC's/UC's to follow.
- ☐ Area Commanders and on-scene IC's/UC's reach agreement on division of responsibility (i.e., media relations, stakeholder meetings, etc.).

AC Planning Chief
- ☐ Provide reporting requirements, formats and time frames.
- ☐ Collect incident IAP's and/or 201's.

AC Logistics Chief
- ☐ Provide procedures for ordering specialized or critical resources.
- ☐ Explain process for sharing or re-assigning specialized and critical resources.
- ☐ Explain demobilization of specialized and critical resources.

AC Finance/Admin Chief
- ☐ Explain process for cost tracking.
- ☐ Explain notification procedures for responder illnesses, injuries or accidents.

On-scene Incident Commanders/UC's
- ☐ Provide overall situation report for their individual incident.
- ☐ Identify resources at risk.
- ☐ Specify current incident objectives.
- ☐ Provide response priorities.
- ☐ Provide long-term projections and existing and anticipated problems.
- ☐ Provide list of resource requirements and shortfalls.
- ☐ Identify probability of success if resource needs are met.
- ☐ Identify consequences if resource requirements are not met.
- ☐ Identify for Area Commanders, areas that AC can provide assistance to them

The diagram shows the following process flow:

AC Staff Meeting → Develop Operating Guide → AC Approve Operating Guide

AC/UC Meeting → Brief Operating Guide

Meeting with IC's/UC's → Monitor Mission Progress → New Ops Cycle Begins

Initial Activities:
- Check-in, AC Briefing & Establish ACP
- Activate AC Organization
- Executive Briefing

AC IC/UC MEETING AGENDA

1. AC PC brings meeting to order, conducts role call, And reviews agenda.
2. AC's provide opening remarks along with providing policy direction, Executives' expectations, AC interim operating procedures, expectations and ground rules.
3. AC PC provides guidance on information reporting to include timeframes, units of measure and formats along with critical information reporting.
4. AC LC provides guidance on ordering and sharing of specialized and critical resources, including demobilization of these resources.
5. AC FC provides guidance on cost accounting and reporting of injuries and accidents.
6. IC's/UC's report on their individual situation to include resources at risk, incident objectives, incident priorities, resource requirements and consequences if resource requirements are not met.
7. Resolve oustanding issues or concerns.
8. AC PC solicits final comments and adjourns the meeting.

AREA COMMANDERS MEETING – During this 1-hour meeting, the AC(s) will use the information derived from the IC meeting and develop overall strategies, objectives, priorities and identify any critical resource needs or issues AC will have to deal with. As needed, AC's will prioritize among incidents. AC(s) will also finalize the AC operating procedures.

When: As soon as possible after adjournment of IC/UC meeting
Facilitator: AC Planning Chief
Attendees: Area Commanders, AC Planning Chief, other staff upon AC request

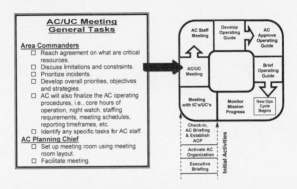

AREA COMMANDERS MEETING AGENDA

1. AC PC brings meeting to order.
2. AC addresses any policies, limitations and constraints.
3. AC reaches agreement on criteria for identifying critical resources.
4. AC discusses and prioritizes incidents.
5. AC PC facilitates discussion and develops overall response priorities.
6. AC PC leads discussion on development of strategic objectives.
7. AC will also finalize the AC operating procedures, i.e., core hours of operation, night watch, staffing requirements, meeting schedules, reporting timeframes, etc.
8. AC identifies any specific tasks for AC staff.
9. AC addresses any critical issues derived from the IC/UC Meeting or Agency Executive Briefing.

AC STAFF MEETING/BRIEFING – During this 1-hour meeting, the AC(s) will present their decisions and management direction to the AC staff. This meeting should clarify and help to insure understanding among

13-31

AREA COMMAND   AREA COMMAND

the core AC staff as to decisions, objectives, priorities, procedures and functional assignments (tasks) that the AC has discussed and reached agreement.

When: Following AC meeting
Facilitator: AC Planning Chief
Attendees: Area Commanders and AC staff to include Unit Leaders and Technical Specialists, if needed

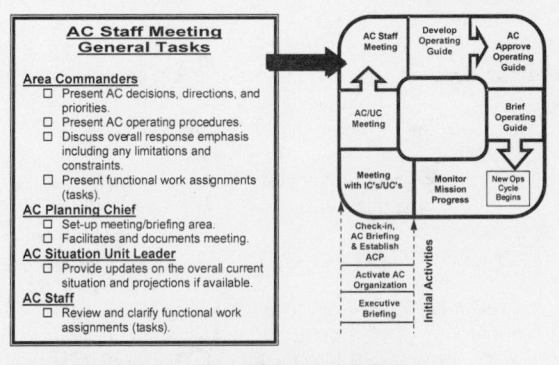

AC Staff Meeting General Tasks

Area Commanders
- ☐ Present AC decisions, directions, and priorities.
- ☐ Present AC operating procedures.
- ☐ Discuss overall response emphasis including any limitations and constraints.
- ☐ Present functional work assignments (tasks).

AC Planning Chief
- ☐ Set-up meeting/briefing area.
- ☐ Facilitates and documents meeting.

AC Situation Unit Leader
- ☐ Provide updates on the overall current situation and projections if available.

AC Staff
- ☐ Review and clarify functional work assignments (tasks).

AC STAFF MEETING/BRIEFING AGENDA

1. AC PC brings meeting to order, conducts role call, covers ground rules and reviews agenda.
2. AC SITL conducts situation status briefing.
3. AC provides comments.
4. AC presents
   a. Decisions, directions, and priorities.
   b. Operating procedures.
   c. Overall response emphasis, including limitations and constraints.
   d. Functional work assignments (tasks) to staff members.
5. AC PC facilitates a short discussion on issues and concerns and adjourns meeting.

DEVELOP OPERATING GUIDE – During this block of time, AC staff develops components that are to be included in the Operating Guide. These components must meet the deadlines set by the PC so Planning can assemble the Operating Guide. Deadline must be early enough to permit timely AC review, approval and duplication.

When: Following AC staff meeting
Facilitator: Planning Chief facilitates process
Attendees: None. This is not a meeting but a period of time.

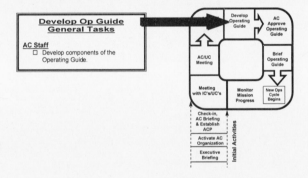

OP GUIDE COMPONENTS	PRIMARY RESPONSIBILITY
1. AC Priorities & Objectives (ICS AC202-CG)	AC CRESL
2. AC Organization List/Chart (ICS AC207-CG)	AC CRESL
3. Critical Resource Summary (ICS AC215-CG)	AC CRESL
4. AC Meeting & Briefing Schedule (ICS AC230-CG)	AC SITL
5. AC Communication Plan (ICS AC205-CG)	AC COML
6. Information Management Plan	AC PIO
7. Critical Information Reporting	AC SITL
8. AC Staffing Schedule	AC CRESL
9. AC Policies, Procedures & Decisions	AC PC

OPTIONAL COMPONENTS (Use as Pertinent)

1. Air Operations Summary (ICS 220-CG)	AC AVSP
2. AC Demobilization Plan	AC PC
3. AC Facility Safety Plan	AC SOFR
4. AC Security Plan	AC SCSP
5. Other AC Plans or documents as required	AC Staff

AC APPROVE OPERATING GUIDE – During this block of time, AC PC assembles Operating Guide, reviews content, makes adjustments if necessary, and provides to AC for review and approval. Following approval duplicates required copies for distribution.

When: Following Operating Guide Development
Facilitator: PC and AC facilitates process
Attendees: None. This is a block of time

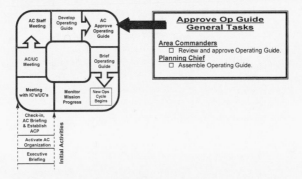

BRIEF OPERATING GUIDE – This 30-minute or less briefing presents the Operating Guide to the AC staff and on-scene IC's/UC's. Briefing to on-scene IC's/UC's may be accomplished by video conferencing or some other medium. Copies are either faxed or sent electronically to on-scene IC's/UC's and Agency Executives.

When: At or as close as possible to AC shift change

Facilitator: AC Planning Chief

Attendees: All AC staff and if possible On-scene IC's/UC's, and Agency Executives

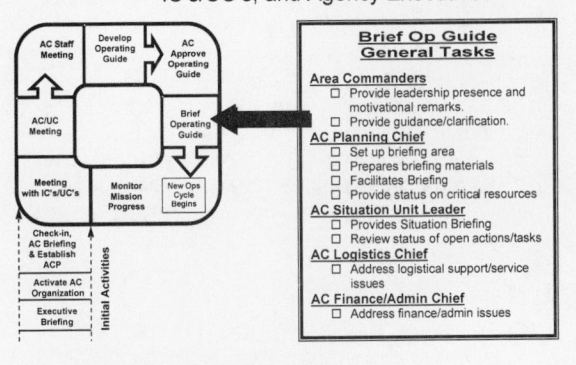

OPERATING GUIDE BRIEFING AGENDA

1. AC PC opens meeting, conducts role call and reviews agenda.
2. AC SITL conducts situation status briefing and provides projections as needed.
3. AC provides opening remarks.
4. AC PC presents Operating Guide.
5. AC LC presents status of specialized and critical resources.
6. AC FC presents status of cost tracking and other cost accounting issues.
7. AC PC conducts round robin to clarify and resolve open issues with participants.
8. AC PC adjourns briefing.

MONITOR MISSION PROGRESS – Assessment is an on-going continuous process to help determine needed adjustments to the operating guide and assist in planning future support to the on-scene operations. Following the AC Operating Guide briefing, and shift change, all AC staff will review mission progress and make recommendations to the AC(s). This feedback/information is continuously gathered from various sources.

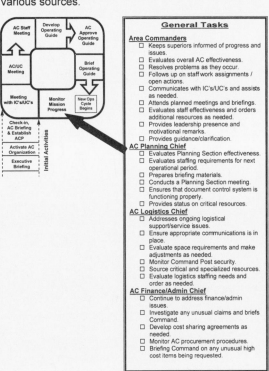

General Tasks

Area Commanders
- ☐ Keeps superiors informed of progress and issues.
- ☐ Evaluates overall AC effectiveness.
- ☐ Resolves problems as they occur.
- ☐ Follows up on staff work assignments / open actions.
- ☐ Communicates with IC's/UC's and assists as needed.
- ☐ Attends planned meetings and briefings.
- ☐ Evaluates staff effectiveness and orders additional resources as needed.
- ☐ Provides leadership presence and motivational remarks.
- ☐ Provides guidance/clarification.

AC Planning Chief
- ☐ Evaluates Planning Section effectiveness.
- ☐ Evaluates staffing requirements for next operational period.
- ☐ Prepares briefing materials.
- ☐ Conducts a Planning Section meeting.
- ☐ Ensures that document control system is functioning properly.
- ☐ Provides status on critical resources.

AC Logistics Chief
- ☐ Addresses ongoing logistical support/service issues.
- ☐ Ensure appropriate communications is in place.
- ☐ Evaluate space requirements and make adjustments as needed.
- ☐ Monitor Command Post security.
- ☐ Source critical and specialized resources.
- ☐ Evaluate logistics staffing needs and order as needed.

AC Finance/Admin Chief
- ☐ Continue to address finance/admin issues.
- ☐ Investigate any unusual claims and briefs Command.
- ☐ Develop cost sharing agreements as needed.
- ☐ Monitor AC procurement procedures.
- ☐ Briefing Command on any unusual high cost items being requested.

13-37

THIS PAGE INTENTIONALLY LEFT BLANK

CHAPTER 14

JOINT FIELD OFFICE
AND
INCIDENTS OF NATIONAL SIGNIFICANCE

References:
  (a) National Response Plan (NRP)
  (b) National Incident Management System (NIMS)
  (c) Joint Field Office Standard Operating Guide (SOP)
  (d) Alignment with the National Incident Management
      System and National Response Plan,
      COMDTINST 16000.27 (series)

NOTE: This chapter provides a very brief overview of
the National Response Plan (NRP), Incidents of National
Significance (INS), and activation of the Joint Field
Office (JFO). For more information and more detailed
guidance, please see references (a) through (d).

INTRODUCTION

For a potential or actual Incident of National Significance
(INS), DHS may establish a Joint Field Office (JFO).
The purpose of a JFO is to provide support to local
Incident Command structures and coordinate efforts to
address broader regional impacts of the incident. As
part of the Multi-agency Coordination System (MACS),
the JFO does not supplant the on-scene Incident
Command(s)/Area Command(s), but supports and
provides broader coordination of incident-related
activities. Execution of tactical operations and
coordination remains the responsibility of the
IC(s)/AC(s).

Activation of a Joint Field Office

When DHS determines that a JFO is necessary, DHS will identify agencies with primary responsibility for incident management to serve a part of the JFO Coordination Group. The JFO Coordination Group will coordinate (usually by teleconference) to define situationally appropriate requirements for a JFO. DHS tasks Emergency Support Function (ESF) #5 (led by FEMA) to stand up a JFO and provide core staffing. Other agencies provide additional staffing of the JFO based on the nature of the incident, typically through the activation of various ESF's. The Principal Federal Official (PFO), PFO Support Staff, and other Senior Federal Officials (SFO's) may operate from an Interim Operating Facility (IOF) until a fully functional JFO is established.

Responsibilities of the JFO Coordination Group

The JFO Coordination Group is comprised of the PFO, who serves as the Secretary of Homeland Security's local representative and agencies with primary responsibility for incident management, such as FEMA's Federal Coordinating Officer (FCO). For incidents that fall largely in Coast Guard jurisdiction, the Coast Guard will participate in the JFO Coordination Group as a SFO. The JFO Coordination Group is responsible for:

a. Overall coordination of Federal incident management and assistance activities across the spectrum of prevention, preparedness, response, and recovery.

b. Ensuring the seamless integration of Federal activities in support of and in coordination with State, local, and tribal organizations.

c. Providing needed resources as requested by the Incident Command and/or relevant EOC's.

d. Providing strategic guidance to Federal entities.

e. Facilitating interagency conflict resolution as necessary.

f. Serving as a primary, although not exclusive, point of contact for Federal interface with State, local, and tribal senior elected/appointed officials, the media, and the private sector.

g. Providing real-time incident information to the Secretary of Homeland Security through the HSOC and the IIMG.

h. Coordinating response resource needs between multiple incidents as necessary.

i. Coordinating the overall Federal public communications strategy locally to ensure consistency of Federal interagency communications to the public.

j. Ensuring that adequate connectivity is maintained between the Incident Command structures; JFO; HSOC; local, county, State, and regional EOC's; nongovernmental EOC's; and relevant elements of the private sector.

Organization of the Joint Field Office

Although the JFO is not an Incident Command structure, it uses an Incident Management Team (IMT) organization to facilitate the integration of multi-agency staffing, provide a robust structure and process for coordinating its activities, and provide a planning cycle for the development of a Coordination Plan. The JFO organization adapts to the magnitude, complexity and nature of the incident. The following diagram is an example JFO organization for natural disasters. For terrorist incidents, the FBI's Joint Operations Center (JOC) is incorporated as a branch within the Operations Section. Likewise, for National Special Security Events (NSSE's), the US Secret Service Multi-agency Command Center (MACC) is also incorporated as a

14-3

branch within Operations. See chapter 23 for more info about NSSE's.

Example JFO Organization for Natural Disasters

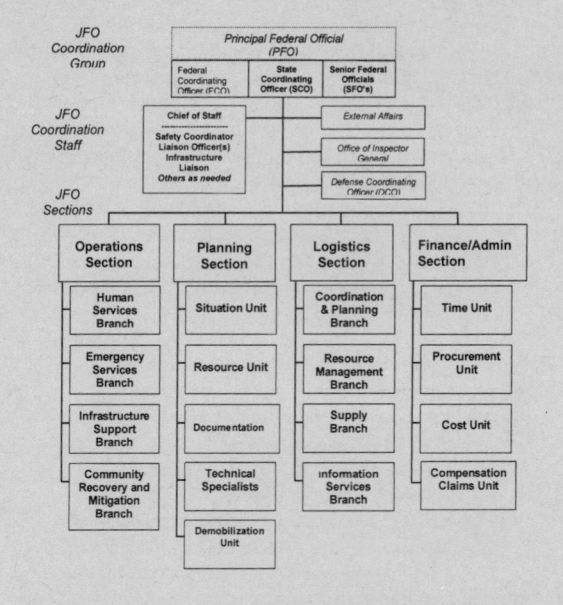

Note: Depending on the magnitude of the disaster, a PFO may not always be designated, in which case the FCO will provide the Federal lead.

The SCO represents the State, and in some instances, the JFO Coordination Group may include local and/or tribal representatives as well as NGO and private-sector representatives, as appropriate.

Coordination between the Incident Command and Joint Field Office

In a response where there is no federal presence in the Unified Command, the JFO primarily works with the involved State EOC's to provide federal assistance. In situations where there is a federal presence in the Unified Command (such as terrorist incidents and oil/hazmat releases), the JFO will coordinate directly with the Unified Command/Area Command. For an effective response, the JFO and the on-scene Incident Command must work together in a cooperative environment. Coordination will take place both at the senior level (i.e., between the Unified Command and JFO Coordination Group) and at the staff levels (e.g., between ICP Planning Section and the JFO Planning Section, Safety Officer and Safety Coordinator, etc.). Based on the incident objectives and Incident Action Plan established by the Unified Command, the JFO establishes broader objectives and creates a Coordination Plan. While developing the broader objectives and Coordination Plan, the JFO Coordination Group must also consider the national strategy and concerns of the Interagency Incident Management Group (IIMG). The Coordination Plan includes objectives established by the JFO Coordination Group, synopsis of agency and Incident Command actions, assigned coordination activities, information-sharing procedures, and a safety plan.

Facilitation Between the JFO and Unified Command

To facilitate cooperation, the on-scene Unified
Command should provide to the JFO:
  a. Incident Priorities.
  b. Copy of Incident Action Plan (IAP) per operational
     period.
  c. Progress updates with identified hindrances.
  d. Critical needs/Critical resource shortfalls (and
     impact of not receiving required resources).
  e. Political, social, economic, and environmental
     impacts.
  f. Long term projections.
  g. Contact directory.
  h. Meeting schedules.

In turn, the JFO:
  a. Provides requested resources.
  b. Coordinates broader objectives with those
     established by the UC.
  c. Addresses resource and policy issues raised by
     the UC.
  d. Synchronizes planning cycle with UC planning
     cycle, as appropriate.
  e. Distributes an overall contact directory.
  f. Provides copy of the Coordination Plan.

14-6

CHAPTER 15

TERRORISM

CHAPTER 15

TERRORISM

References:
  (a) National Response Plan (NRP)
  (b) National Incident Management System (NIMS)
  (c) Coast Guard Hazmat Response Special Teams
      and Capabilities Contact Handbook
  (d) U.S. Coast Guard Maritime Law Enforcement
      Manual (MLEM), COMDTINST 16247.1 (series)

INTRODUCTION

A nuclear, biological, or chemical Weapon of Mass
Destruction (WMD) type terrorist incident is inherently a
hazardous substance incident. As such it should be
responded to under the National Response System
(NRS). As applicable, consult Chapter 20 Hazardous
Substance (Chemical, Biological, Radiological and
Nuclear) and Chapter 22 (Multi-Casualty) of this
Incident Management Handbook (IMH) regarding
establishment and use of the Incident Command
System when a terrorist incident precipitates a
hazardous materials release and/or mass casualty.

The UC responding to an incident where terrorism is
involved have to be acutely aware of the unique nature
of the Federal Government's response mechanism for
these types of incidents. All agencies must use the
National Plan (NRP) structures and the National
Incident Management System (NIMS) to coordinate all
Federal assistance to State and local governments for
response activities to Incidents of National Significance
(INS). During a terrorism incident, the UC may work for
the Federal Bureau of Investigation (FBI) and/or FEMA
and will be guided by the NRP

15-2

If an incident occurs without warning that produces major consequences and appears to be caused by an act of terrorism, then FEMA and the FBI will initiate response actions concurrently. FBI will have the lead in this incident because of the possible terrorism link and all agencies will be guided by the NRP.

With the exception of the U.S. Coast Guard National Strike Force (NSF), upon notification of WMD/Terrorism incident, USCG policy is to stay clear of the contaminated area and to provide command, control and support only. NSF Strike Teams are the only units within the Coast Guard who are currently trained and have a mission to respond to chemical incidents for either Coast Guard or the U.S. Environmental Protection Agency (USEPA) Federal On-Scene Coordinators. For personnel responding to WMD/Terrorism events, certain guidelines should be followed:

- Hesitate – don't rush in and ask questions later! Take time to decide what to do.
- Evaluate the situation – size up the situation - think about what's happening and what you should do.
- Isolate – after evaluating where the hot zone is, don't let anyone other than a responder enter the hot zone, and don't let other responders enter the hot zone without proper equipment. Set up a barrier line, even if you have only simple yellow emergency tape.
- Evacuate – get people out of the hot zone without risking your own life. Don't go into the hot zone without proper equipment. Keep victims and others who might have been exposed from getting too far away – medical and police will want to talk to them.

15-3

- Decontaminate – but only if you can do it without endangering yourself. Use a fire hose if possible so you won't have to get close to the victims; in some cases a victim can self decontaminate.
- Cooperate – when other responders arrive, follow standard organizational principles. But above all cooperate; there'll be time later to argue who's boss; right now try to save lives.
- Communicate – let other emergency and medical authorities know what your situation is and what you're doing. But if you think there might be a flammable vapor around, don't use your radios (or any other electrical equipment) near the incident. Retreat to a vapor free area to use that radio.
- Investigate – actually, the first responder won't do any real criminal investigation, but you must remember this is a crime scene and responders and others shouldn't disturb crime scenes. Preserve the crime scene (for all terrorism is a crime as well as an act of war); observe, remember, and report to police.
- Be aware of possible secondary devices, including explosive, radiological, chemical and biological. Be cognizant of surroundings, especially of containers, or packages that appear misplaced. A tactic terrorist's use involves setting off a device designed to draw in first responders and then setting off a secondary device to maximize casualties.
- Ask qualified authorities, typically the FBI, if the area has been cleared of secondary devices.
- Again, be aware that in a WMD incident terrorists generally have a singular purpose and that is to cause fear, death and destruction. A defensive stance should always be maintained for a WMD incident.

15-4

TERRORISM INCIDENT SPECIFIC NIMS ICS POSITIONS AND TASK DESCRIPTIONS

Only those ICS positions and tasks specific and unique to Terrorist Incident missions will be described in this section. Persons assigned the common positions consistent with the NIMS organization should refer to position job aids and Chapters 5 through 11 of this Manual for their position/task descriptions and checklists.

INCIDENT COMMANDER - Tasks specific to a Terrorist Incident are to:

    a. Review Incident Commander responsibilities in Chapter 6.

    b. Assesses the need for additional resources and assist in obtaining their assistance. Some of these resources are listed in the Terrorism Special Teams section of this chapter.

    c. Ensure that the following have been established:

- HAZMAT Group – which is responsible for deploying a reconnaissance team, produce sampling/identification, assisting with victim rescue, setting up decontamination for responders and developing a plan of action for containment and control of hazardous agents.
- Medical Group – which is responsible for initiating victim rescue, patient decontamination, and emergency medical care for NBC victims.
- Hospital Coordination – which establishes communication links with area hospitals, provides them with situation reports, and information on agent identification, and determines pharmacology needs.

- Medical Information & Research – which begins to research agent characteristics based upon victim signs and symptoms, victims' descriptions of agent, sample characteristics, and other information as it becomes available. Establishes communication with Poison Control Centers (ATSDR and CDC).
- Law Enforcement Group – which coordinates law enforcement agencies to establish incident security, establishes evidence collection and control, and obtains intelligence information.

d. Work to identify and address strategic and tactical issues.

e. Work with city and county mental health resources to assure that Critical Incident Stress Management services are provided to victims, their families, first responders, and the general public.

f. Coordinate with the County Medical Examiner/Coroner to establish appropriate forensic and mortuary services for deceased victims.

g. Assist the Safety Officer in establishing a site safety plan; implementing an accountability system; and establishing hot, warm, and cold zones if not already established.

PUBLIC INFORMATION OFFICER - Tasks specific to a terrorist incident are:

a. Review Public Information Officer Responsibilities in Chapter 6.

b. Establish safe media conference areas distant from the Incident Command Post.

c. During the Event:

1. Determine what information is appropriate to

15-6

release to avoid panic.

2. Promote optimum community response.
3. Develop information releases that support response activities:
   - Medical treatment sites that the victims can report to.
   - Transportation avenues and other areas that are closed off.
   - Immediate first aid measures that can be taken.
   - Location of shelter facilities where evacuated personnel have been moved to.

d. After the Event:
1. Release non-sensitive information.
2. Provide basic information regarding the event:
   - Where, what, why, how.
   - Units responding.
   - Number of casualties.
3. Examples of types of information that should not be released:
   - Names of fatalities.
   - Specific type/name of agent involved (until after incident is terminated).
   - Dispersal method(s) used.
   - Specific law enforcement activities.
   - Condition of victims.

EVENT SITE BRANCH DIRECTOR - Tasks specific to terrorist incidents are:
a. Review Branch Director Responsibilities in Chapter 7.
b. Coordinate for site control around the vicinity where the event occurred.
c. Determine hazards presented by the event (monitoring/detection).

    d. Establish a safe refuge and a casualty collection area.

    e. Establish emergency decontamination capability.

    f. Coordinate with Medical Unit for medical treatment and transport capability, including requesting county transit buses.

    g. Coordinate with Safety Officer for a site safety and control plan.

    h. Determine containment and control procedures to be used.

    i. Coordinate with other agencies (investigative/ evidence gathering).

COMMUNITY IMPACT BRANCH DIRECTOR - Tasks specific to terrorist incidents are:

    a. Review Branch Director Responsibilities in Chapter 7.

    b. Coordinate for perimeter security and traffic control.

    c. Determine hazards presented to the community through detection/monitoring.

    d. Determine best protective actions to use:
   - Rescue
   - Shelter-in-place (SIP)
   - Evacuation
   - Establish shelters

    e. Establish emergency decontamination capability for off site personnel and public.

    f. Establish a medical treatment and transport capability for off-site personnel and the public.

    g. Coordinate with Safety Officer for site safety and control plan.

    h. Coordinate with Information Officer to develop emergency broadcast messages to alert and update the community.

    i. Determine re-entry procedures to be used

j. Coordination with other agencies and notify the County Health Officer.

HAZARDOUS SUBSTANCE/MATERIALS GROUP -
Tasks specific to terrorist incidents are:
  a. Review the Division/Group Supervisor Responsibilities in Chapter 7.
  b. Review the Chemical tasks in Chapter 19 of this document.
  c. Ensure the implementation of defensive mitigation practices when indicated.
  d. Ensure that information regarding the agent(s) and patient symptoms is passed to the Medical Group.
  e. Ensure patients are properly decontaminated.

MEDICAL GROUP - Tasks specific to terrorist incidents are:
  a. Review Common Responsibilities in Chapter 2.
  b. Direct medical care delivery to response personnel and incident victims.

HOSPITAL COORDINATION UNIT - The Medical
Group usually performs these responsibilities and duties, but this unique unit is established to assist at terrorist incident responses. Their tasks are:
  a. Review Unit Leader Responsibilities in Chapter 2.
  b. Serve as liaison for local medical facilities receiving patients.
  c. Ensure vital incident management information is communicated to each receiving hospital.
  d. Provide the medical communities with the needed patient care information for the agent(s) involved, in cooperation with the Technical Specialist-Medical Information & Research.
  e. Implement a system of patient tracking in concert with the on-scene EMS personnel and facilities

receiving patients.

f. When requested, serve as clinical consultants to the medical staff at each medical facility-receiving patients by providing advice on patient care, personnel safety, or facility protection, in cooperation with the Technical Specialist-Medical Information & Research.

TECHNICAL SPECIALIST-MEDICAL INFORMATION & RESEARCH - The Medical Group performs these responsibilities in collaboration with National Response Center (NRC), an emergency communication infrastructure designed to assist Federal responses to incidents.

a. Identify needed research materials that will assure optimum access to the most current, complete, and accurate information available on nuclear, biological, or chemical (NBC) agents.

b. Perform the research needed to identify the agent(s) involved, physical characteristics, appropriate PPE, and information about possible signs and symptoms to be observed, treatments to be initiated, antidotes to be utilized, and possible long-term effects. This activity will be completed by assimilating information from several sources including:
   - Technical Specialist-Reference & Resources in the Hazardous Substance Group.
   - Regional Poison Control Center.
   - CHEMTREC.
   - Various special teams listed on page 15-14.

c. Communicate vital mitigation and clinical management information to the Medical Group including:
   - Needed patient care information for the agent(s) involved.

15-10

- Antidote needs of each facility and assist them in obtaining the needed items from the regional cache, government agencies, or vendors. Serve as clinical consultants to the medical staff at each facility receiving patients, by providing advice on patient care, personnel safety, or facility protection.

LAW ENFORCEMENT GROUP - Tasks specific to terrorist incidents are:

a. Review Division/Group Supervisor Responsibilities in Chapter 7.
b. Review Law Enforcement Group Tasks in Chapter 17 of this Manual.
c. Review Appendix J of reference (d).
d. Obtain pertinent law enforcement information in order to coordinate the operational response from the following:
   - FBI field office.
   - Local law enforcement agencies.
   - State law enforcement/traffic agencies.
   - Local fire and rescue agencies, including HAZMAT teams.
   - Local Emergency Operations Centers.
   - Pertinent NBC information discussed at intelligence sharing forums.
   - Current national and international events involving terrorist group activities.
   - Intelligence from all sources.
e. Advise the IC of law enforcement related issues and latest intelligence information.
f. Be familiar with local law enforcement resources available (Bomb Squads, etc.).
g. Assist in obtaining needed resources from law enforcement operations.
h. Assure incident security issues are identified and

addressed.

i. Verify the incident. Determine if a terrorist act has occurred.

j. Respond to the scene with sufficient personnel to address the incident.

k. Initiate appropriate callback of additional personnel as needed.

l. Establish inner and outer perimeters, based on the nature of the incident.

m. Provide security for the Command Post.

n. Verify the identification of the responding personnel.

o. Coordinate incident site evacuation.

p. Coordinate evacuation of surrounding areas as needed.

q. Coordinate traffic flow, especially ingress and egress of emergency/rescue

r. Provide evidence identification, collection and control, including:

- Establish control and protection of the crime scene.
- Coordinate the collection/preservation of evidence with the FBI.
- Mapping/photographing of all evidence locations.
- Collection of non-contaminated evidence.
- Coordination of collection, chain of custody, and safe storage of contaminated evidence with the Hazardous Substance/HAZMAT Group.
- Provide secure, safe storage for collected evidence.

s. Affect the arrest and transportation of the perpetrators when possible.

MEDICAL TECHNICAL SPECIALIST (Planning Section) - The Medical Group usually performs these responsibilities and duties, but this unique position is established to assist at terrorist incident responses in the planning section. This position (preferably filled by a physician) is responsible for:

   a. Review Common Responsibilities in Chapter 2.
   b. Review Medical Group tasks in Chapter 19 of this manual.
   c. Serve as medical advisor to the Incident Commander and Operations Section Chief.
   d. Develop and implement the medical action plan in conjunction with the Medical and Hazardous Substance/HAZMAT Groups.
   e. Assure effective liaison with local EMS agencies and medical facilities.
   f. Perform additional tasks and duties as assigned during an incident.

MENTAL HEALTH COORDINATION - First responders will receive Critical Incident Stress Management services through departmental resources. Victims, their families, and the general community will receive Critical Incident Stress Management services through established sources, including the Airport Chaplains, American Red Cross Disaster Mental Health Services and County Mental Health Services.

CORONER COORDINATION - The City/County Medical Examiner/Coroner staff, according to the Mass Casualty Incident Plan, will process deceased victims once the FBI has released the scene. The City/County Examiner/Coroner will assist the law enforcement branch with collecting evidence from deceased victims upon request. Federal mortuary resources are also available, if requested.

TERRORISM INCIDENT TECHNICAL TEAMS

Resources for a WMD/Terrorism incident response are similar to that of a chemical incident response. The NIMS ICS should be followed and the State and local responders who normally respond to a chemical incident will also respond to a WMD incident. However, the FBI should be notified during a WMD event, and due to the extreme nature of a WMD incident, DOD resources may also be needed.

The FBI is the lead agency for a WMD incident. If upon arriving on scene and USCG personnel suspect the incident to be WMD related, the FBI and NRC should be contacted through proper channels. FEMA is also a lead agency under the NRP to support the incident response.

There are several Special Teams that have response capabilities for WMD/Terrorism incidents and are listed in more detail in reference (c), Coast Guard Hazmat Response Special Teams and Capabilities Contact Handbook which can be found at the following website: http://homeport.uscg.mil/ and are listed here:

- Agency for Toxic Substances and Disease Registry (ATSDR) Emergency Response Teams
- U.S. Marine Corps Chemical Biological Incident Response Force (CBIRF)
- Department of Energy Nuclear Emergency Support Team (DOE NEST)
- USEPA Environmental Response Team (EPA ERT)
- USEPA Office of Enforcement, Compliance, and Assurance (OECA), National Counter-terrorism Evidence Response Team (NCERT)

- USEPA Radiological Emergency Response Team (EPA RERT)
- Federal Bureau of Investigation, Laboratory Division, Hazardous Materials Response Unit (FBI HMRU)
- National Oceanic and Atmospheric Administration Office of Response and Restoration (NOAA OR&R) Hazardous Materials Response Division (HAZMAT)
- USCG National Pollution Funds Center (USCG NPFC)
- USCG National Strike Force (USCG NSF)
- Occupational Safety and Health Administration Health Response Team (OSHA HRT)
- United States Navy (USN) Supervisor of Salvage and Diving (SUPSALV)
- United States Army Corps of Engineers Rapid Response Program (USACE RR)
- Department of Defense (DOD) Joint Director of Military Support (JDOMS)
- Department of Homeland Security (DHS), Federal Emergency Management Agency, Metropolitan Medical Response System (MMRS)
- USEPA Diving Program
- USEPA Emergency Communications and Outreach Team (ECOT)
- USEPA Emergency Response Peer Support and Critical Incident Stress Management (Peer Support/CISM) Team
- USEPA Ocean Survey Vessel, Peter W. Anderson
- United States National Guard Civil Support Teams (USNG CST)

THIS PAGE INTENTIONALLY LEFT BLANK

CHAPTER 16

Maritime Security/Antiterrorism

CHAPTER 16

MARITIME SECURITY/ANTITERRORISM

References:
(a) Maritime Security/Antiterrorism Job Aid
(b) National Response Plan (NRP)
(c) National Strategy for Maritime Security (NSMS)
(d) National Maritime Transportation Security Plan (NMTSP)
(e) Maritime Transportation Security Act of 2002 (MTSA)
(f) Coast Guard Strategic Plan for Combating Terrorism – Maritime Sentinel
(g) National Response Options Matrix (NROM)
(h) 33 CFR Subchapter H – Maritime Security
(i) Navigation and Vessel Inspection Circular (NVIC) 9-02
(j) Public Law (PL) 106-390/42 U.S.C. 5121, et seq. The Robert T. Stafford Disaster Assistance and Emergency Relief Act
(k) Reimbursement from the Federal Emergency Management Agency (FEMA), COMDTINST 7300.8 (series)
(l) Maritime Infrastructure Recovery Plan (MIRP)
(m) Critical Incident Communications, COMDTINST 3100.8 (series)

INTRODUCTION

Maritime Security. Maritime security, as used in this Chapter, refers to Area Maritime Security (AMS) antiterrorism measures (i.e., prevention and defensive-oriented protection) that are used to reduce the vulnerability of the Marine Transportation System (MTS), individuals and property to terrorist acts, to include limited response and containment by local

16-2

forces. Maritime security/antiterrorism also includes immediate measures for initial MTS support response and thereafter to facilitate recovery required to reestablish MTS functions, and cargo flow in particular. Maritime security antiterrorism activities for the MTS and its components are continuously conducted from pre-incident through incident response and through immediate recovery actions to completion of recovery operations in order to deter or prevent multiple incidents, to protect critical maritime infrastructure, and to support MTS recovery. Law enforcement (LE) and counterterrorism aspects of maritime security are addressed in Chapters 15 and 17. Where LE or counterterrorism response is required during incident management, AMS antiterrorism measures are a supporting activity.

Please see the Maritime Security/Antiterrorism Job Aid, reference (a), for more information.

Continuing Antiterrorism Requirement During Incident Management. Antiterrorism security requirements are a continuing responsibility during incident management in support of references (b) through (f), and must be effectively represented, coordinated, and conducted regardless of the initiating hazard or cause of an incident. An incident that occurs which is or threatens to become a Transportation Security Incident (TSI) triggers prearranged enhanced antiterrorism security measures within the affected area to protect the MTS, with emphasis on critical maritime infrastructure. Such an event would likely also result in the Commandant, U.S. Coast Guard, implementing additional security measures, as well as changes in maritime security (MARSEC) and force protection levels within the MTS but outside of the area that is immediately impacted by the incident. This action would be guided by reference (g) and the known elements of the incident.

An incident that begins as other than a security event may nevertheless require enhanced antiterrorism security measures to protect the MTS. These measures are in addition to force protection measures. During incident management, enhanced local antiterrorism security measures may also be mandated from the national level in response to another incident in another location or through proactive changes in MARSEC levels. The maritime security component of antiterrorism, as discussed below, must be incorporated into the operations and planning sections of the incident command structure.

Maritime Security Activities. A maritime security framework with antiterrorism measures that respond to mandated requirements and a risk-based management strategy has been established for each port area within that area's Maritime Transportation Security Act (MTSA)-mandated Area Maritime Security Plan (AMSP) per references (e), (h) and (i).

Maritime Security (MARSEC) Levels. Maritime security emphasis is governed by MARSEC levels that are set by the Commandant, U.S. Coast Guard, in coordination with the Department of Homeland Security. The Commandant sets the MARSEC level consistent with the Homeland Security Advisory System (HSAS) and that Threat Condition's scope of application. The Commandant retains the discretion to adust the MARSEC level when necessary to address particular security concerns or circumstances related to the marine transportation system. The lowest MARSEC level, MARSEC 1, is generally comparable with the level of risk associated with HSAS Threat Levels LOW

16-4

through ELEVATED (GREEN/BLUE/YELLOW) , thereby accommodating the continually higher baseline level of risk associated with marine operations. This correlation reflects the continually higher baseline level of risk associated with marine operations. The Coast Guard Sector Commander, serving as Coast Guard Captain of the Port (COTP), has been delegated authority to unilaterally increase the local MARSEC level under exceptional circumstances according to criteria contained in reference (k).

AREA MARITIME SECURITY

Area Maritime Security (AMS). AMS under MTSA, reference (e), and implementing regulations, reference (h), and covers the full preparedness continuum of prevention, protection, response, and recovery and develops details, measures, procedures and strategies for preventing and responding to a TSI, and facilitating recovery of the MTS after a TSI. AMS activities are coordinated locally by the Coast Guard Captain of the Port (COTP) as the Federal Maritime Security Coordinator (FMSC). Actual operations and responses are conducted under applicable organization, community-based and incident-specific operating, contingency and response plans, as available.

AMS During Incident Management. AMS provides an existing local maritime security foundation, including coordination and communications arrangements with the port community for initiating incident management by a unified command for a large-scale local transportation emergency, Transportation Security Incident (TSI), or Incident of National Significance. An incident in any of these categories could originate from or involve one or a combination of hazards including terrorism, natural disaster, civil disturbance, or

16-5

oil/hazardous material spill. Consequently, it is essential to correlate and coordinate the continuing and enhanced AMS activities across ICS groups (e.g., Maritime Security, Law Enforcement (LE), Oil and Hazardous Materials, Search and Rescue (SAR), and MTS Response and Recovery) and maritime-related support of Emergency Support Functions (ESF).

AMS activities at MARSEC 1 provide a framework and pre-established coordination and communications arrangements for providing prevention and protection of maritime resources during an incident, initiating incident management for local marine transportation security emergencies, and supporting prevention and protection for effects of other emergencies. Facility and vessel-specific security plans also provide critical information to support response to an incident involving one or more of these assets. Maritime security and marine safety activities also provide some of the core and supporting resources in varying degrees of capability for responding to any category of hazard affecting the MTS, and within the immediate area around ports and waterways. Immediate MTS recovery activities within the impacted area also provide essential elements of information (EEI) needed by the Coast Guard, Customs and Border Patrol (CBP), Transportation Security Administration (TSA), and Department of Transportation (DOT) to facilitate recovery and restoration of cargo flow outside of the impacted areas per reference (l).

Area Maritime Security Committee (AMSC). Preparedness is co-developed with port stakeholders. Preparedness activities include formation and coordination of Area Maritime Security Committees selected per criteria in reference (i); identification of critical port infrastructure and operations; identification of risks (threats, vulnerabilities, and consequences)

16-6

through risk-based assessments; determination of mitigation strategies and implementation methods; development and description of the process by which to continually evaluate overall port security; preparation of AMS plans including details of additional security measures for increases in MARSEC levels, incident unified command, response and recovery structure, responsibilities and capabilities, procedures for security response and for facilitating MTS recovery. The AMSC provides planning and coordination support; it is not considered a response entity for the purposes of crisis management..

Area Maritime Security Plans (AMSP). Antiterrorism measures are enumerated in AMSPs, which are supported by facility-specific and vessel-specific security and response plans. These plans are designated as Sensitive Security Information (SSI) and are restricted from public access. The AMSPs are supporting plans to references (a), (c), (e), (h) and (j). Plan content is specified by reference (i). <u>An AMSP is not a first responder plan, but an awareness, preparedness and prevention plan as well as a supporting plan for response and MTS recovery</u>. AMSP development considers possible roles, responsibilities, and resources very broadly and is generally limited to determining who will respond, what their roles will be, what resources they can provide, and procedures that they will use. The AMSP provides a framework for communication and coordination amongst port stakeholders and law enforcement and public officials to:

- Identify and reduce vulnerabilities to security threats in and near the MTS.
- Implement special procedures to ensure marine safety, and the safety and readiness of personnel, installations, and equipment,

- Coordinate implementation of prevention and protection procedures during response, and
- Facilitate and support coordinated MTS recovery and restoration activities.

AMS planning is supported or supplemented on a port-by-port, case-by-case basis by local plans and other materials (e.g. underwater port security plans, maritime counterterrorism plans, response and recovery job aids). AMSPs and Area Contingency Plans (ACP) for oil and hazardous materials typically involve many of the same stakeholders, and may be implemented concurrently based on the prevailing circumstances.

MTS Recovery This section addresses measures that are needed within the area impacted by a TSI to provide initial recovery and to provide the basis to facilitate long-term recovery and mitigation activities as characterized below:

- <u>Initial Recovery</u> – MTS infrastructure has been returned to service and is capable of operations at some level. Activities, policies or mitigation strategies aimed at recovery are considered to be achievable in 90 days or less.
- <u>Long-term recovery</u> – MTS infrastructure has been returned to pre-incident condition or has the capacity to operating at pre-incident levels. Activities, policies or mitigation strategies aimed at long-term recovery may take longer than 90 days. Generally parallels long-term recovery measures associated with Emergency Support Function (ESF) #14.

The Coast Guard is responsible for recovery of agency infrastructure and for MTS infrastructure that it directly administers (e.g. aids to navigation). Sector

Commanders, as Captains of the Port (COTP) and FMSC, are responsible for developing coordinated initial recovery activities in consultation with AMSCs for MTS infrastructure that is subject to references (d) and (g). MTS recovery should also be coordinated with mitigation measures covered by ACPs that are related to the MTS.

MARITIME SECURITY-ANTITERRORISM SPECIFIC NIMS ICS POSITIONS AND TASK DESCRIPTIONS

Only those ICS positions and tasks specific and unique to Maritime Security antiterrorism responsibilities will be described in this section. Persons assigned the common positions consistent with the NIMS organization should refer to position job aids and Chapters 5 through 11 of this Manual for their position/task descriptions and checklists.

Area Maritime Security includes immediate operational measures as well as planning for security and recovery operations. Area maritime security antiterrorism is addressed in the Operations Section. MTS security and recovery activities are planned in the Planning Section and conducted through the Operations Section.

INCIDENT COMMANDER - Tasks specific to an Incident are to:

a. Review Incident Commander (IC) responsibilities.
b. Review Maritime Security responsibilities as delineated in AMSPs.
c. Determine HSAS threat level and MARSEC level and required maritime security measures.
d. Determine if unilateral local-area increase in MARSEC level is necessitated by the incident.
e. Comply with critical incident communications requirements in reference (m)
f. Ensure that the following have been established:
   - Maritime Security Group in Operations Section – which coordinates implementation of MARSEC measures, coordinates maritime security activities with the law enforcement (LE), oil and hazardous materials, search and rescue (SAR), and MTS recovery groups.
g. Implement supporting plans as applicable.

16-10

    h.   Work to identify and address tactical and strategic issues.

    i.   Assist the Coast Guard component commander in coordinated maritime security and MTS response and recovery operations and activities consistent with the AMSP, site safety plan, law enforcement, oil and hazardous materials, and search and rescue operations.

    j.   Determine antiterrorism support required for military outloads in or through the affected area.

AREA MARITIME SECURITY GROUP - Tasks specific to security incidents are:

    a.   Review the Division/Group Supervisor Responsibilities in Chapter 7.

    b.   Coordinate implementation of MARSEC levels changes.

    c.   Monitor and report attainment of MARSEC measures and deficiencies, ensuring the implementation of MARSEC requirements.

    d.   Assist the Incident Commander in meeting critical incident communications requirements of reference (m).

    e.   Implement AMSP contingency arrangements and procedures.

    f.   Coordinate AMS oversight and support with AMSC.

    g.   Coordinate AMS support for LE, oil and hazardous materials, SAR and MTS recovery activities.

    h.   Coordinate implementation of supporting plans (e.g. underwater port security).

    i.   Arrange for, document and report MTS damage assessments.

    j.   Coordinate AMS support for MTS Recovery.

    k.   Coordinate AMS support for ESF activities.

    l.   Coordinate AMS support for military outload

operations in or through the affected area.

MTS RECOVERY UNIT - Tasks specific to recovery of the MTS are:
   a. Review MTS Unit Leader responsibilities in Chapter 8.
   b. Activate MTS recovery unit assist team (where available).
   c. Be familiar with the AMSC and AMSP and associated recovery procedures and priorities. .
   d. Identify and implement supporting MTS recovery plans, where available.
   e. Incorporate MTS security and recovery into ICS planning cycle.
   f. Advise the IC and PSC of maritime security issues associated with MTS recovery and latest EEI from port community stakeholders in coordination with the Maritime Security, LE, oil and hazardous materials and SAR Groups.
   g. As needed, assist IC, PSC and OSC in prioritization of critical infrastructure needed to be brought to operational status.
   h. Determine and advise the IC and PSC of relevant pre-scripted FEMA mission assignments under the Stafford Act, reference (j), related to or required for MTS recovery.
   i. Coordinate with IC, PSC, FEMA and pertinent ESFs for FEMA/Stafford Act mission assignments through the Joint Field Office (JFO) in support of MTS response to reestablish a basic capability for long-term recovery.
   j. Assess and advise IC and PSC of unified command capability to perform any FEMA mission assignment requests received through the JFO.
   k. Coordinate with the LE Group to determine the relationship of evidence protection requirements

to recovery operations.

l. Identify short and long term issues affecting or potentially affecting the MTS with supporting materials.

m. Identify supporting requirements.

n. Review and apply as applicable reference (k) recommendations for MTS Recovery.

o. For incidents impacting more than one Coast Guard Sector, provide information to support management of regional issues, including local area impacts that will be felt outside of the immediate response area, such as export delays.

p. Make recommendations to the IC and PSC on short term (impact felt within 90 days) recovery priorities and actions.

THIS PAGE INTENTIONALLY LEFT BLANK

CHAPTER 17

LAW ENFORCEMENT

CHAPTER 17

LAW ENFORCEMENT

References:
  (a) U.S. Coast Guard Maritime Law Enforcement
      Manual (MLEM), COMDTINST 16247.1 (series)
  (b) Maritime Counter Drug and Alien Migrant
      Interdiction Operations Manual, COMDTINST
      M16247.4 (series)
  (c) National Response Plan (NRP)
  (d) National Incident Management System (NIMS)

INTRODUCTION

The organization for a major Law Enforcement
Operation (Counter Drug or Alien Migrant Interdiction) is
designed to show an organizational structure that could
provide supervision and control for the essential
functions required during such an operation.

It must be emphasized that this guide is not a substitute
for law enforcement planning as outlined in the
references (a) and (b). The Commandant and Area
manuals, operation orders and policies that could
include plans for such major multi-agency/multi-nation
that would lead major Counter Drug or Alien Migrant
Interdiction Operations should identify the organizations,
resources, and command and control structure that
would be utilized in the operation. Exercising these
plans will develop and fine-tune national and agency
roles in the IC/UC and ICS.

The normal law enforcement action for Coast Guard
units will be single unit activities. Reference (b)
identifies the structure for these normal single unit
operations and dictates in detail how the operation is to

be carried out. Since NIMS ICS is the primary system used by most Federal, State, and Local government agencies, and is required by references (c) and (d) to be used in response to incidents, it is advantageous to use and understand the ICS process in a large multi-agency and multi-national operation where the incident brings numerous agencies together with overlapping jurisdictions, responsibilities, and capabilities. In these situations, Coast Guard Law Enforcement personnel may be expected to fill Command and General Staff positions, with other agencies in the role of IC an/or within an UC. In this IMH, the goal is to build upon the structure identified in reference (b), and demonstrate how the IC/UC and ICS organization may be used when a Law Enforcement Operation grows from a single unit operation to a Multi-Agency/Multi-National Operation.

For example, an alien migrant interdiction operation such as the Mariel Boat Lift can generate a huge multiple-agency response with a limited command and control structure. Because the Coast Guard is usually the first unit on-scene and because of its mission responsibilities and capabilities, it will be instrumental in building the final overall command and control team.

Although there are many types of law enforcement activities, a major multi-agency Alien Migrant Interdiction Operation was selected to demonstrate how the expanding modular ICS organization might be used to manage a Law Enforcement Operation. Commandant and Area instructions, manuals and operation orders include references, plans and policies that dictate overall U.S. Coast Guard Law Enforcement operations policy. For example, OPLAN VIGILANT SENTRY provides the overall Department of Homeland Security response to a mass migration in the Caribbean.

LAW ENFORCEMENT ACTIVITY SCENARIO AND MODULAR ORGANIZATION DEVELOPMENT

MODULAR DEVELOPMENT - A series of examples of modular development are included to illustrate one method of expanding the ICS organization.

INITIAL RESPONSE ORGANIZATION - A U.S. Coast Guard cutter is on normal patrol when it intercepts a small boat fitting the profile of an undocumented migrant vessel. The Coast Guard cutter carries out the standard boarding operation procedures for the vessel. See Page 17-7 for an example of the Initial Response Organization.

REINFORCED RESPONSE ORGANIZATION - Upon boarding the profiled vessel, the boarding party discovers a large number of undocumented migrants. During the boarding party's search and investigation, the interpreter overhears one of the undocumented migrants express his concern for relatives aboard another vessel. The Commanding Officer of the cutter relays this information to the U.S. Coast Guard District with operational control over his mission, and a Coast Guard aircraft is deployed to search for the other vessel. The District Commander assumes the role of lead agency and IC for the interdiction operation, and requests the appropriate U.S. Coast Guard Area Commander to direct an additional cutter to his operational control to assist in the search for other possible undocumented migrant vessels. The District Commander also notifies local DOD units that there is a possibility of additional undocumented migrant vessels in the operational area. The second cutter has additional Law Enforcement Detachments (LEDETs) assigned before sailing. See Page 17-8 for an example of the Reinforced Response Organization.

MULTI-DIVISION/GROUP ORGANIZATION - Within a day of searching, the Coast Guard aircraft and JIATF resources have identified numerous vessels of all sizes that fit the undocumented migrant vessel profile. This information is relayed to the District, who in turn notifies the Area Commander and Coast Guard Headquarters. Coast Guard Headquarters notifies the Immigration and Customs Enforcement (ICE) and other federal law enforcement agencies. Upon notification to these agencies by Coast Guard Headquarters, the Commandant will normally give authorization for direct communication to the District Commander. The Area Commander orders all available cutters (WHEC, WMEC) to the area for interdiction operations under the operational control of the District Commander. DOD lends its resources to assist in the search for undocumented migrant vessels. See Page 17-9 for an example of the Multi-Division/Group Organization.

The Department of Homeland Security assigns a representative to assist and coordinate its activities with the District Commander. The District Commander's Staff and Agency Representatives are tasked with developing the resource requirements for the extended interdiction operation, and determining the resources that will have to be obtained from outside the District. The District Chief of Operations is assigned as the OSC. The operational area is divided into geographical divisions and a Coast Guard cutter is assigned to each division for patrol and boarding operations. A Navy vessel is directed to the scene to serve as an undocumented migrant holding area. ICE provides aircraft for additional search patrols.

Since many of the vessels being used to carry undocumented migrants are sailing under the flag of other nations, the U.S. Coast Guard has requested through the Department of State that representatives of those governments be assigned as ship riders to Coast Guard vessels, allowing them to carry out boardings on the applicable nations vessels in international waters.

The IC/UC establishes a JIC to handle the intense media interest that is developing over the operation.

MULTI-BRANCH ORGANIZATION - As the situation develops, the number of undocumented migrants discovered and detained by the Coast Guard has grown beyond the capability of vessels to safely and humanly hold them offshore. The IC/UC has determined that holding facilities must be prepared on shore. The IC/UC identify Federal, State and Local resources to assist in planning and implementing the shoreside facilities. See Page 17-10 for an example of the Multi-Branch Organization.

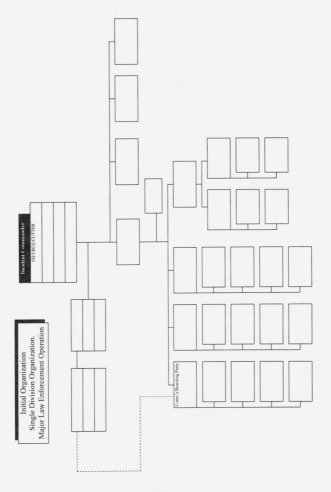

LAW ENFORCEMENT

LAW ENFORCEMENT

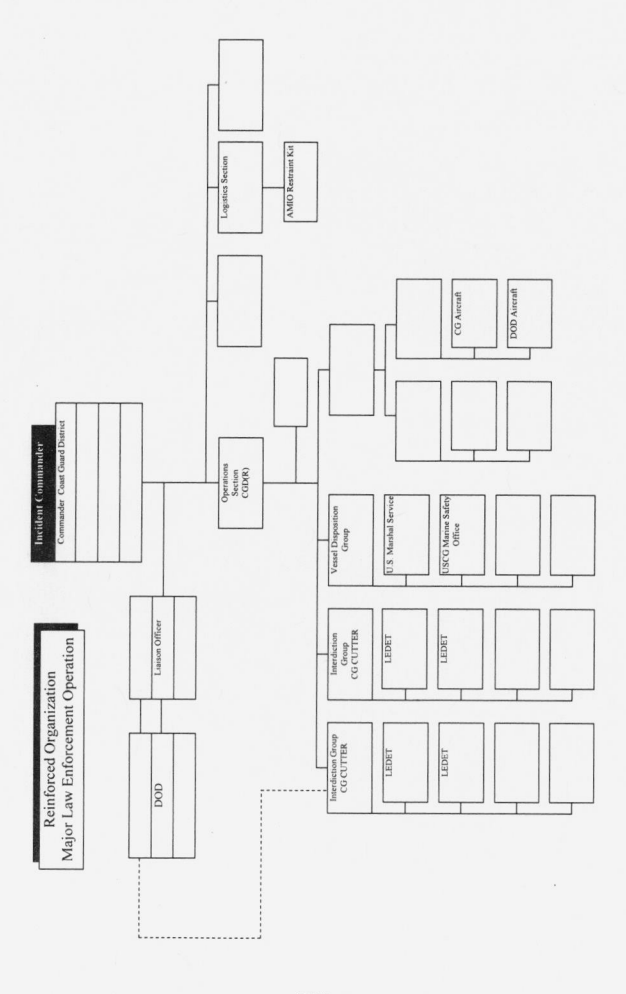

**Reinforced Organization
Major Law Enforcement Operation**

LAW ENFORCEMENT   LAW ENFORCEMENT

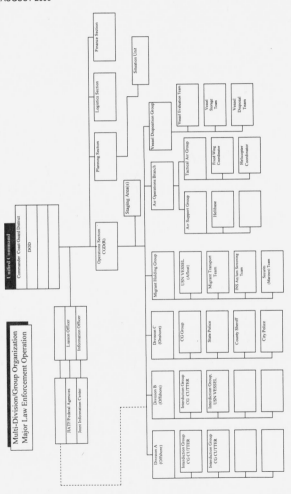

LAW ENFORCEMENT　　　　LAW ENFORCEMENT

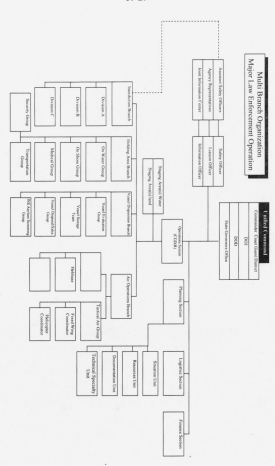

Multi Branch Organization
Major Law Enforcement Operation

Unified Command
- Commander Coast Guard District
- DOJ
- DOD
- State Governors Office

- Assistant Safety Officers
- Agency Representatives
- Joint Information Center

- Safety Officer
- Liaison Officer
- Information Officer

Operations Section (CGOPA)

Planning Section

Logistics Section

Finance Section

Interdiction Branch
- Division A
- Division B
- Division C
- Security Group
- On Water Group
- On Shore Group
- Medical Group
- Transportation Group

Holding Area Branch

Vessel Disposition Branch
- Vessel Evaluation Group
- Vessel Storage Team
- Vessel Disposal/Sales Group
- INS Asylum Screening Group

Staging Area(s) Water
Staging Area(s) land

Air Operations Branch
- Helibase
- Tactical Air Group
  - Helicopter Coordinator
  - Fixed Wing Coordinator

- Situation Unit
- Resources Unit
- Documentation Unit
- Technical Specialty Unit

LAW ENFORCEMENT ACTIVITY SPECIFIC ICS POSITIONS AND TASK DESCRIPTIONS

Only those ICS positions and tasks specific and unique to Law Enforcement missions will be described in this section. Persons assigned the common positions consistent with the NIMS ICS organization should refer to position job aids and Chapters 5 through 11 of this IMH for their position/task descriptions and checklists.

ASYLUM PRESCREENING OFFICER (APSO) - The APSO is responsible for conducting initial screenings of individuals who have made asylum claims or come from a nation with a history of political persecution, human rights violations, or torture. APSOs are full time asylum officers deployed to the field. The APSO will normally be assigned to the LO as an Agency Representative or directly to the Command Staff.

These prescreening interviews determine if an individual has a credible fear of persecution upon return to his/her home nation. APSO interviews are transmitted to CIS Headquarters in Washington, D.C., for review by asylum specialists. If it is determined that an individual has a credible fear of persecution, the person is taken to another location for more extensive interviews. While the APSO may be assigned in various locations within the ICS, he/she needs to have direct access to communications with Washington, D.C. The contents of APSO interviews may be confidential and not available for intelligence or general use. Additional duties include:

a. Review the Agency Representative Responsibilities in Chapter 6.
b. Advise the IC/UC on the procedures for asylum interviews, specific support required, and the separation of those claiming asylum.

    c.   Liaise with CIS Headquarters on asylum issues.

    d.   Conduct additional interviews as necessary.

    e.   Advise the IC on trends in asylum claims and indicators that those within the IC/UC may need to be aware of.

VESSEL DISPOSITION GROUP SUPERVISOR - The Vessel Disposition Group Supervisor is responsible for the disposal of vessels seized in the course of Law Enforcement Operations. In some cases this will involve warning the return of the vessel to the flag state, but in many situations the vessel will be seized for forfeiture (either because it is stateless or because it was used in the commission of a crime). In drug interdiction missions, this task is usually performed by Immigration and Customs Enforcement (ICE). In all other cases, the U.S. Marshal Service performs this function.

If an asset is seized for forfeiture, all hazardous materials must be removed and all safety violations must be corrected before the vessel can be disposed of. The lead agency will contract out for removal and disposal of hazardous materials from the vessel using private contractors. U.S. Coast Guard Sectors may be asked to assist the lead agency in assessing the condition of the vessel, the applicable environmental laws that may apply to the vessels condition, and steps needed to correct the assessed violations. Addition duties included:

    a.   Review the Division/Group Supervisor Responsibilities in Chapter 7.

LAW ENFORCEMENT DETACHMENT TEAM
LEADER - Law Enforcement Detachment Team (LEDET) Leaders are responsible for separate teams of individuals trained in boarding vessels for conducting law enforcement operations. LEDETs typically deploy to U.S. Navy and foreign naval vessels to provide them with law enforcement capability. They can also be used in various situations to augment Coast Guard Cutter Boarding Teams, and in these cases should not be confused with the Cutter's Boarding Team, which is made up of individuals permanently assigned to the Cutter's crew. Addition duties included:
   a. Review the Strike Team Leader/Task Force Responsibilities in Chapter 7.

MARITIME SAFETY AND SECURITY TEAMS -
Maritime Safety and Security Teams (MSSTs) were created under the Maritime Transportation Security Act (MTSA) 2002, in direct response to the terrorist attacks on Sept. 11, 2001, and are a part of the Department of Homeland Security's layered strategy directed at protecting our seaports and waterways. MSSTs provide waterborne and a modest level of shoreside antiterrorism force protection for strategic shipping, high interest vessels and critical infrastructure. MSSTs are a quick response force capable of rapid, nationwide deployment via air, ground or sea transportation in response to changing threat conditions and evolving Maritime Homeland Security (MHS) mission requirements. Multi-mission capability facilitates augmentation for other selected Coast Guard missions.

THIS PAGE INTENTIONALLY LEFT BLANK

CHAPTER 18

SEARCH AND RESCUE

TABLE OF CONTENTS

CHAPTER 18

SEARCH AND RESCUE

References:
- (a) IMO/ICAO International Aeronautical and Maritime Search and Rescue Manual, Vols. I & II
- (b) U.S. National Search and Rescue Supplement (NSS) to the International Aeronautical and Maritime Search and Rescue Manual (IMSAR)
- (c) National Search and Rescue Plan, 1999
- (d) U.S. Coast Guard Addendum to the National Search and Rescue Supplement (NSS) to the International Aeronautical and Maritime Search and Rescue Manual (IMSAR), COMDTINST 16130.2 (series)
- (e) National Response Plan (NRP)
- (f) National Incident Management System (NIMS)

INTRODUCTION

Search and Rescue (SAR) efforts primarily focus on finding and assisting persons in actual or apparent distress and are carried out within a well-defined SAR response system as per references (a) – (d). These references have their basis in international law that U.S. SAR services are obligated to follow, and they have practical benefits that are intended to maximize the effectiveness of SAR operations, particularly when working with other military services, SAR authorities of other nations, and with ships or aircraft at sea. When an emergency warrants responses in addition to SAR, the NIMS ICS organizational structure shall be used for overall response management in accordance with reference (e) and (f). Examples of other activities that are not SAR, but are often closely associated with a SAR incident, include search and recovery, salvage,

SEARCH & RESCUE   SEARCH & RESCUE

AUGUST 2006

investigation, fire-fighting, pollution response, etc. This chapter describes an example ICS organizational structure that will provide supervision and control of essential functions during a SAR incident that includes, or will include, non-SAR response activities.

For incidents that actually or potentially involve both SAR and non-SAR response activities, the SAR Mission Coordinator (SMC), who is designated by the SAR response system, will initiate action and coordinate the overall SAR response in accordance with references (a) through (d). When the Incident Commander (IC) is designated, the SMC function will be placed under the umbrella of the ICS organizational structure, typically as the SAR Branch Director or SAR Group Supervisor in the Operations Section. Simply put, the SAR response system "plugs into" the ICS organizational structure, where the SMC (or someone designated by the SMC to carry out this function) serves as the "plug" or link. The SAR response may also include a SAR On-Scene Coordinator (SAR OSC) and an Aircraft Coordinator (ACO). In some cases the person serving as the Incident Commander (IC) or Operations Section Chief (OSC) may also be designated as the SMC, but the terms "Incident Commander" or "Operations Section Chief" are not interchangeable with titles associated with SAR response functions. For the majority of incidents, the SAR response will be completed/suspended by the time the ICS structure is fully in place. As the SAR mission winds down and other missions take precedence (i.e., search and recovery), the IC may designate the SMC or SAR OSC in the SAR response system to continue as a Branch Director or Group Supervisor in the ICS structure to manage on-scene operations other than SAR. Likewise, Search and Rescue Units (SRUs) may also be reassigned to other groups in the ICS structure once the SAR mission is concluded. In general, Coast Guard

18-3

personnel with SAR responsibilities should receive
sufficient ICS training to enable them to carry out their
respective duties in ICS response organizations.

SEARCH AND RESCUE BEST RESPONSE

KEY AREAS TO A SUCCESSFUL SAR RESPONSE

Success of response operations can often be found in
how well the management team focused on key
response areas. ICs and their Command and General
Staff should consider, if applicable, the following key
response areas during ICS activation in conjunction with
or following a search and rescue operation.

OPERATIONAL	SUPPORT/COORDINATION
Search Planning & Operations	Safety
Rescue Planning & Operations	Stress Management
Medical/Triage	Liaison with Victim's Families
Fire Fighting	Security
Shoreline Search & Recovery	Investigations
On-Water Search & Recovery	Resources
	Political
	Assisting & Cooperating Agencies
	Public Information
	Command Post Needs

IC's and their Command and General Staff need to
closely monitor how well the incident objectives,
strategies, and tactics are addressing the key response
areas identified above and adjust, as necessary, to
ensure the maximum potential for the best possible
response.

SEARCH AND RESCUE INCIDENT SCENARIO
AND MODULAR ORGANIZATION DEVELOPMENT

MODULAR DEVELOPMENT - A series of examples of modular development are included to illustrate one method of expanding the major airline crash incident organization.

INITIAL RESPONSE ORGANIZATION (MAJOR AIRLINE CRASH) - The SAR Mission Coordinator (SMC), initiates emergency response actions and designates the best-qualified and most capable unit on-scene as SAR OSC. The SMC may also designate an ACO to manage air assets on-scene if there are too many for the SAR OSC to effectively manage or communications between surface and air assets prove challenging. The first to arrive on scene would likely be USCG vessels and aircraft, police/fire boats, fishing vessels, and hosts of recreational boats. The FAA will be requested to establish air space restrictions and issue the appropriate Notice to Airmen (NOTAMs). The cognizant Sector Commander or District Commander may be designated the IC, at which time the SMC function is placed under the umbrella of the ICS organizational structure. Rescue and emergency medical treatment will take priority during this phase. Recovery and identification of the deceased, accident investigation, and cleanup will take priority later in the incident. Initial responders will be heavily involved in the rescue, triage, and transportation of survivors. A PIO is immediately assigned to provide initial information to the media and establish a JIC. CERT and/or CISM support should be considered early. See Page 18-9 for an example of the initial response organization.

REINFORCED RESPONSE ORGANIZATION (MAJOR AIRLINE CRASH) - An ICP is established and initially staffed with personnel from the Coast Guard; local, state, and federal law enforcement and emergency response/management agencies; and local medical institutions/organizations. The JIC should be staffed for 24-hour operations, if need be. A LNO is also designated to coordinate the large numbers of responding and interested government agencies and public organizations. The SOFR is assigned to assess the safety hazards/situation and develop a Site Safety Plan (ICS-208). The NTSB and the FBI may be added to the UC upon their representative's physical arrival on-scene. See Page 18-10 for an example of the reinforced response organization.

The Operations Section Chief (OSC) is designated to manage the growing number of operational activities (e.g., SAR, medical care, security, and evidence collection). This may be the Sector Commander if the District Commander assumes the role of IC. The following Groups are established to organize the operational activities:

- The SAR Group continues to carry out the SAR response under the function of the SMC. Additional surface and air assets have arrived from different jurisdictions. Tactical control of some or all of the response assets may be shifted to the SAR Group for tasking by the SAR OSC or ACO.
- The Medical Group, supported heavily by local EMS and hospital personnel and resources, coordinates triage and treatment areas, as well as transporting survivors. A Patient Transportation Unit may be established to efficiently move survivors from the staging/triage areas to medical facilities.
- The Law Enforcement Group begins the task of

securing the scene; providing shore-side security for staging areas and the ICP, establishing evidence collection and control; and conducting the investigation. If criminal activity is not suspected, the NTSB may have primary investigative responsibilities. If terrorism is suspected, the FBI will take the lead. NTSB and FBI representatives will participate in the UC and brief the UC concerning their needs regarding investigation and recovery operations. A Traffic Control Unit may be needed to keep tremendous number of shore-side curiosity seekers from impairing the access of EMS/rescue personnel to critical Staging Areas.

- An Air Tactical Group Supervisor may be designated to coordinate assignments and air assets and manage air tactical activities.
- Consideration should be given to establishing a Demobilization Unit.

MULTI-DIVISION/GROUP ORGANIZATION (MAJOR AIRLINE CRASH) - The UC and Command Staff are functional and fully staffed. The District may be designated as the Coast Guard IC to be on the same level as the NTSB and FBI representative(s). The Sector Commander may assume the role of OSC, if he or she has not already done so. Deputies from the fire, law enforcement, and emergency medical service agencies could assist the OSC. The Rescue, Medical, and Law Enforcement Groups are fully developed. The rescue is nearly complete, if not already completed, and the operation is shifting to search and recovery of bodies and aircraft debris. Surface and air assets are shifted to other groups, such as the Search and Recovery and Law Enforcement Groups. See page 18-11 for an example of the Multi-Division/Group Organization.

18-7

The focus of the UC's efforts is shifting to the NTSB and law enforcement agencies, including city/county/state coroner. A Body Recovery Team has been added and is working closely with the coroner who has jurisdiction. An Underwater Recovery Group has been initiated and may be led by the Navy or other qualified agencies. The FBI, NTSB and local/state law enforcement agencies are coordinating the investigation and recovery of wreckage.

The JIC continues to be fully staffed. Additional assets may be needed to accommodate the political dignitaries and next of kin that would want to view the accident site or have direct briefings from the Command Staff.

MULTI-BRANCH ORGANIZATION (MAJOR AIRLINE CRASH) - The UC is fully functional and staffed. UC efforts are focused on NTSB and FBI concerns. The Coast Guard is now primarily assisting with search and recovery activities, as well as providing host/landlord support. The appropriate deputies and assistants have been designated to ensure an integrated and coordinated operation at the Section, Branch, Division, and Group levels. See Page 18-12 for an example of the Multi-Branch Organization.

The recovery operation has been divided into three branches (i.e., Surface, Underwater, and Shore-side). Geographic divisions have been created to divide the search and recovery into manageable areas.

Although not shown on the organization chart, a Demobilization Unit may be established in the Planning Section to develop an Incident Demobilization Plan. This plan should include the Chaplain and/or CISM.

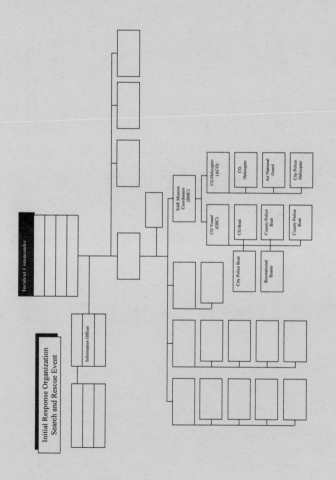

Initial Response Organization
Search and Rescue Event

Incident Commander

Information Officer

SAR Mission Coordinator (SMC)

CG Vessel (OSC)

CG Helicopter (ACO)

CG Boat

City Police Boat

County Police Boat

Recreational Boater

County Police Boat

CG Helicopter

Air National Guard

City Police Helicopter

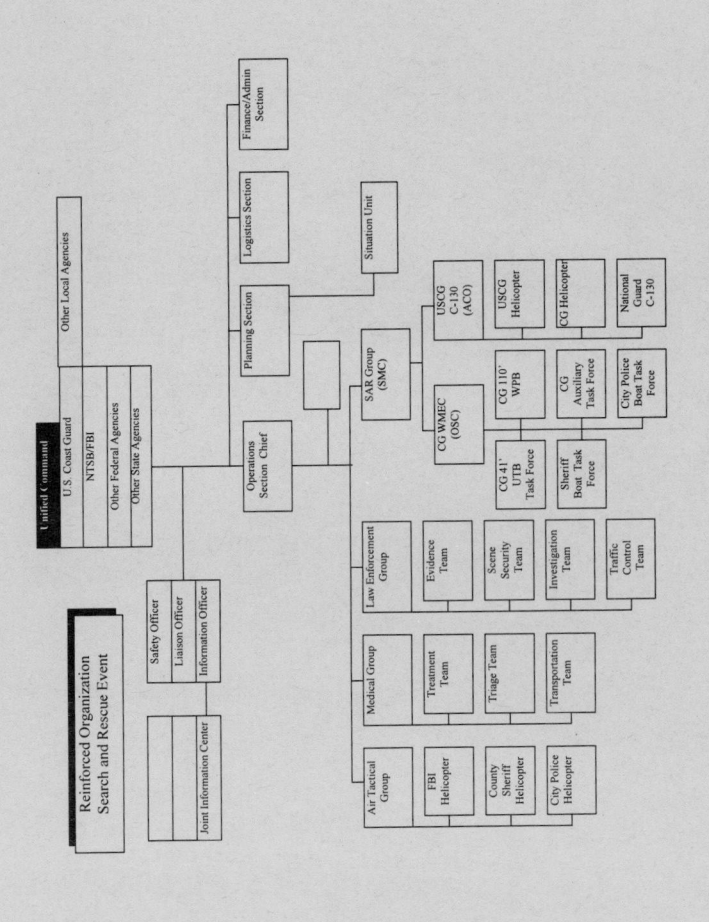

Reinforced Organization Search and Rescue Event

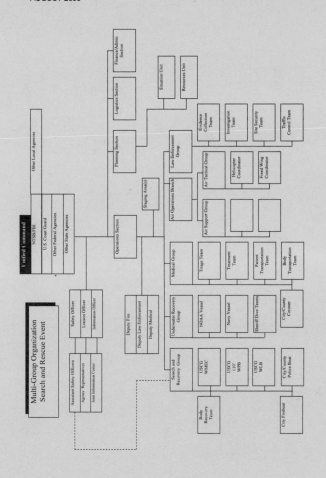

Multi-Group Organization
Search and Rescue Event

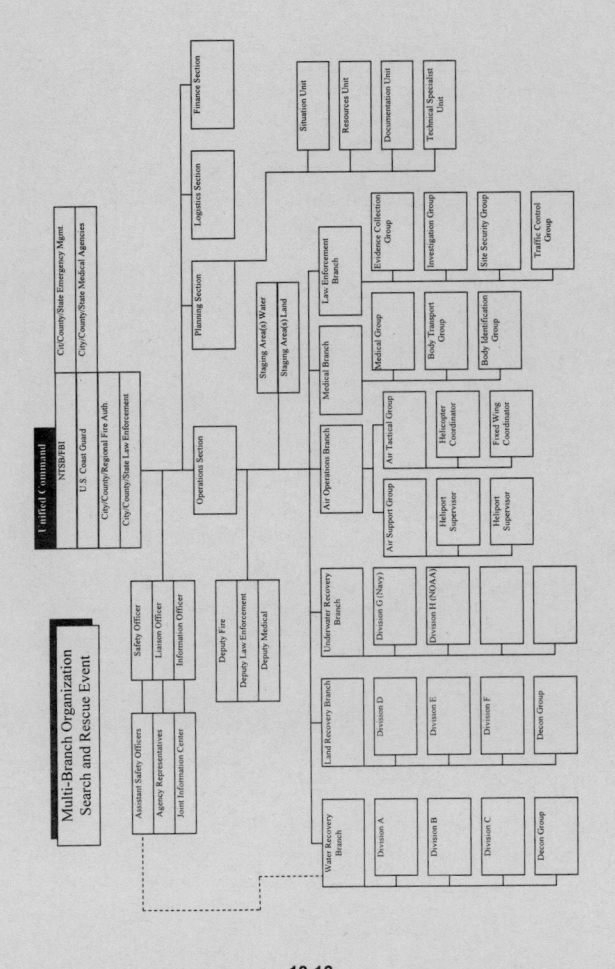

Multi-Branch Organization
Search and Rescue Event

SEARCH & RESCUE   SEARCH & RESCUE

SEARCH AND RESCUE SPECIFIC ICS
POSITIONS AND TASK DESCRIPTIONS

Only those ICS positions and tasks specific and unique to Search and Rescue (SAR) missions will be described in this section. A general description of SAR Response System Specific functions is also included. Persons assigned the common positions consistent with the NIMS ICS organization should refer to the position job aids and Chapters 5-13 of this IMH for their position/task descriptions and checklists.

INCIDENT COMMANDER (IC) - In addition to the responsibilities outlined in Chapter 2, the IC (and the OSC if one is designated) of an incident that includes a SAR mission must recognize that the SAR Mission Coordinator (SMC) is obligated to carry out the SAR mission in accordance with references (a) – (d). The SMC (or someone designated by the SMC for this function) serves as the link between the SAR Response System and the ICS organization and is best placed at the Branch Director or Group Supervisor level (for further description and duties of the SMC, see SAR System Specific Functions below). The IC may also be designated as the SMC; however, separate individuals should carry out the IC and SMC functions if the operational tempo and/or span of control warrant it or the IC is not thoroughly familiar with all SAR system processes. For SAR incidents that actually or potentially include other non-SAR activities (i.e. search and recovery, salvage, investigation, pollution response, fire-fighting, etc.), carry out the following tasks as appropriate:
  a. Establish a suitable ICP, preferably at a site separate from the OPCEN, and stand-up ICS organization apart from initial response operations.

18-13

- Assign personnel to establish the ICP and stand-up ICS organization <u>that are not responsible for initial response actions</u> (i.e., personnel not coordinating or prosecuting the SAR case).
- Establish an ICP, and accommodate to the best extent possible and as necessary the following four components: (1) at-sea command and control; (2) reconstruction, investigation and human remains transfer (primarily involving mass casualties); (3) family briefings; and (4) media briefings and access.
- Activate/request Incident Management Assist Team (IMAT) augmentation.
- If it is not operationally feasible for the SMC to be physically located at the ICP, the SMC should assign a liaison to the ICP to represent the SMC.

b. Mobilize additional appropriate resources as soon as possible to stabilize the situation or assist in the recovery, salvage, pollution response, firefighting, etc. (i.e., tugs, fireboats, charter boats, salvage vessels, etc.).

c. Have the District Command Center contact the FAA to establish a Temporary Flight Restriction (TFR) for the airspace over the area of incident/operations.

d. Ensure the following Groups are established, if necessary:
- Medical Group to coordinate emergency medical care, including transportation to medical facilities, for Person On Board (POB) of a distressed vessel or craft (descriptions of these functions are found in Chapter 19).

- Law Enforcement Group to coordinate law enforcement agencies to provide shore-side security of Staging Areas and the ICP, establish evidence collection and control, and assist with enforcement of safety and/or security zones (descriptions of these functions are found in Chapter 14).

e. Immediately assign or request a PIO to provide initial information to the media and establish a JIC to provide timely information and updates on progress of SAR efforts and outline of future actions.

- Ensure that the JIC is staffed for 24-hour operations, if necessary, to meet the demands for information by the media, community groups, and public in general.
- Be available, as the IC, to provide press briefings. If the SAR response is on-going, ensure the SMC is aware of all press briefing plans

f. Coordinate with the SMC to notify Next of Kin (NOK) as soon as possible and maintain daily contact with them to provide progress of SAR efforts and outline future actions. The IC shall ensure the greatest possible sensitivity in interacting with family and friends of the victims. Note: For cases involving airline crashes, the airlines are responsible for making NOK notifications.

- For SAR incidents involving large numbers of victims, especially in cases of mass casualties or prolonged searches, ensure that lodging is centrally located and/or easily accessible for those NOK who arrive in the area. This will facilitate daily briefings.

- Establish an area where families of victims can receive daily mission briefings. For incidents involving large numbers of POB, this should be at the place where NOK are centrally lodged.
- If the operational tempo does not allow the IC to provide the NOK briefings personally, assign a senior officer who is disengaged operationally from the SAR incident to provide this as a primary task.
- Provide information on mission progress and future actions to the NOK before releasing it to the media.
- Notify NOK of a decision to suspend SAR efforts prior to suspending search for missing POB.

g. The SMC or SAR Coordinator may continue the SAR mission beyond the time when a case would normally be suspended due to humanitarian considerations, large number of people involved, or forecast of greatly improved search conditions.

However, when the potential for saving life is minimal, Search and Rescue Units (SRUs) will not be put at unnecessary risk. Nor should they continue searching in that situation when their use may preclude their availability for other missions.

NOTE: Only those agencies designated as U.S. SAR Coordinators (i.e., the USCG for maritime regions) have the authority to suspend a SAR case.

h. When scheduling surface and air SRUs, utilize fatigue standards found in Appendix K of reference (d) and applicable policies of the operational commander.

i. For incidents involving firefighting, establish a Firefighting Group to coordinate local authorities responsible for fighting fires on vessels or at waterfront facilities. Note: This should be coordinated prior to an incident. During marine firefighting situations, CG units shall adopt a conservative response posture and focus actions on those traditional Coast Guard activities not requiring CG personnel to enter into a hazardous environment.

- The CG Captain of the Port (COTP) is the USCG entity responsible for coordinating firefighting activities.
- As per reference (d), CG personnel shall not actively engage in firefighting (other than fires on CG vessels) except in support of a regular firefighting agency under the supervision of a qualified fire officer. CG assistance is available only to the degree of training level and adequacy of equipment.
- CG personnel shall not engage in independent firefighting, except to save a life or in the early stages of a fire to avert a significant threat without undue risk.

OPERATIONS SECTION CHIEF (OSC) – In addition to the responsibilities outlined in Chapter 7, the OSC of an incident must recognize that the SMC is obligated to carry out the SAR mission in accordance with references (a) – (d). The OSC may also be designated, and perform the function of the SMC, if operational tempo and/or span of control allow it, and the person is thoroughly familiar with all SAR system processes (for further description and duties of the SMC see SAR Response System Specific Functions below).

SAR SYSTEM SPECIFIC FUNCTIONS

(Note: These functions are provided for information of the IC. SMC's and SAR OSCs are to use established guides and procedures set forth in references (a) - (d) and in standard operating procedures.

SAR MISSION COORDINATOR (SMC) - The SMC is designated (usually pre-designated) by the SAR Response System for each specific SAR mission and coordinates the overall response to a SAR incident in accordance with references (a) – (d). In the U.S. Coast Guard, the SMC designation is done by a responsible Command Center that serves as a Rescue Coordination Center (RCC) or Rescue Sub-Center (RSC). SMC responsibilities typically include:

a. Gathering detailed information relating to the distress situation.

b. Issuing an Urgent marine Information Braodcast (UMIB) to inform mariners in the area of the distress situation and to instruct them to either keep clear of the area or to request their assistance.

c. Conduct SAR operations in accordance with standard SAR procedures and standards as set forth in references (a) – (c).

d. Assign a SAR On-Scene Coordinator (SAR OSC) as appropriate to improve on-scene coordination.

e. Use search planning tools to develop search plans that optimally use available resources.

f. Ensure all documentation from the SAR mission, to include copies of SITREP's, logs, SAR Action Plans, photo/video film, etc., are provided to the Documentation Unit Leader.

SAR On-Scene Coordinator (SAR OSC) - The SAR OSC coordinates the SAR mission on-scene using the resources made available by SMC and should <u>safely</u>

18-18

carry out the SAR Action Plan in accordance with references (a) - (d). The SAR OSC may serve as a Branch Director or Group Supervisor to manage on-scene operations after the SAR mission is concluded and other missions continue, such as search and recovery. SAR OSC responsibilities typically include:

a. Establish and maintain communications with the SMC.
b. Assume operational control and coordination of all SRUs assigned until relieved or mission is completed.
   - Establish and maintain communications with all SRUs using assigned on-scene channels.
   - Require all aircraft to make "operations normal" reports to the SAR OSC.
   - Establish a common altimeter setting for all on scene aircraft.
   - Obtain necessary information from arriving SRU's, provide initial briefing and search instructions, and provide advisory air traffic service to aid pilots in maintaining separation from one another.
c. Carry out SAR action plans.
   - Receive and evaluate all sighting reports, and divert SRUs to investigate sightings.
   - Obtain search results from departing SRUs.
d. Submit sequentially numbered situation reports (SITREPs) to the SMC at regular intervals.

TECHNICAL SPECIALISTS/EQUIPMENT

PARARESCUEMAN (PJ) TECHNICAL SPECIALIST - These members of the USAF are specialists in the rescue, stabilization, and recovery of personnel from remote areas, often under extremely hazardous conditions, including combat. PJs provide emergency medical treatment (at the paramedic level) necessary to stabilize and evacuate injured personnel.

  a. PJ's often provide worldwide search, rescue and recovery assistance associated with aircraft accidents, disaster relief, humanitarian evacuation, and contingency landing support for NASA missions.

  b. If deployed from fixed-wing assets, they jump with a Rigged Alternate Method Zodiac (RAMZ), providing them with a small boat to help facilitate rescues.

FLIGHT SURGEON - The flight surgeon is a physician that has attended a special course that has prepared them to provide medical support in the aviation community. They are qualified to fly or provide medical consultation.

COAST GUARD RESCUE SWIMMER – All Coast Guard Air Stations with helicopters have highly trained helicopter rescue swimmers who are EMT qualified. They are trained to deploy from the helicopter to recover an incapacitated victim from the water, day or night.

SELF-LOCATING DATUM MARKER BUOYS (SLDMB's) – All Coast Guard Air Stations and many Coast Guard surface units and small boat stations are equipped with self-locating datum marker buoys (SLDMB) which can provide high quality, extended duration current information. SLDMB's provide frequent, high-resolution (GPS-based) position information independent of any on-scene unit. Section 4.11 of Ref (d) provides detailed information on SLDMB's.

CHAPTER 19

OIL SPILL

TABLE OF CONTENTS

CHAPTER 19

OIL SPILL

References:
  (a) National Response Plan (NRP)
  (b) National Incident Management System (NIMS)
  (c) National Contingency Plan (NCP)
  (d) NPFC User Reference Guide
  (e) FOSC Field Finance & Resource Management (FFARM) Guide
  (f) Technical Specialist Job Aid

INTRODUCTION

The Coast Guard is a regulatory agency for industries involved in the transport of oil, routinely supports other agencies in their response to oil spills, and may become involved in oil spills when responding or supporting responses to other incidents such as terrorist actions, hazardous materials releases from chemical carriers, accidents at non-transportation related facilities that may be located within a COTP Zone, etc. It is impossible to address the possible ICS organizations that may result from the above scenarios. It is important to note that the majority of oil spills are small events that will not and should not result in a response beyond that of an initial or reinforced response organization. It should also be noted that the capabilities in various COTP zones throughout the country vary greatly. The COTP must have knowledge of the local government response capability and be familiar with the local and state ICs as this will affect the degree of leadership and control that the Coast Guard will be expected to take in oil spill response. In areas where the state and local government have a strong oil spill response program,

19-2

the Coast Guard may be primarily in a support role during the emergency phases. In areas where there is no oil spill response capability, the Coast Guard may be expected to take a much stronger leadership role.

In this regard, there may also be reasons to expand the UC beyond the FOSC, SOSC, and Responsible Party IC (RPIC) participation that has become the standard for oil spill response. The organizations reflect that under OPA 90 regulations, the responsible party (RP) who has had the oil spill is mandated to follow an approved Facility Response Plan (FRP) or Vessel Response Plan (VRP), to provide a spill management team for managing the oil spill, and to become a member of the UC. For a full description of a specific ICS position assignment or task, the reader should refer to the appropriate task assignment provided in Chapters 5 -11.

OIL SPILL BEST RESPONSE
DELIVERING "BEST RESPONSE"

IC's and their Command and General Staffs need to closely monitor how well the incident objectives, strategies, and tactics are addressing "Best Response" and key response functions, and to make appropriate adjustments where necessary to ensure the maximum potential for success.

The term "Best Response" means that a response organization will effectively, efficiently, and safely respond to oil spills, minimizing the consequences of pollution incidents and to protect our national environmental and economic interests.

"Best Response" equals a successful response based on achievement of certain key success factors (i.e. the

things that a response must accomplish to be
considered successful) as follows:

• **Human Health** □ No public injuries □ No worker injuries • **Natural Environment** □ Source of discharge minimized □ Source contained □ Sensitive areas protected □ Resource damage minimized • **Economy** □ Economic impact minimized	• **Public Communication** □ Positive media coverage □ Positive public perception • **Stakeholders Support** □ Minimize stakeholder impact □ Stakeholders well informed □ Positive meetings □ Prompt Handling of claims • **Organization** □ Standard Response Mgmt Syst □ Sufficient/Efficient resources

When conducting an oil spill response, ICs and their
Command and General Staffs should always consider
the "Best Response" concept while managing
operational and support/coordination functions.

OPERATIONAL
Search and Rescue
Fire Fighting
Salvage and Lightering
Protection
Shoreline recovery
On-Water recovery
Dispersants
Assessment
In-Situ Burning
Wildlife
Disposal
Hazardous Substance

SUPPORT/COORDINATION
Public Information
Assisting and Cooperating Agencies
Environmental
Economic
Political
Claims
Natural Resource Damage
Investigations
Safety
Command Post Needs

OIL SPILL   OIL SPILL

OIL SPILL ACTIVITY SCENARIO AND MODULAR ORGANIZATION DEVELOPMENT

MODULAR DEVELOPMENT
A series of examples of Modular Development are included to illustrate one method of expanding the Incident Organization at an oil spill incident. The examples shown are not meant to be restrictive, nor imply that these are the only ways to build an ICS organizational structure from an initial response to a multi-branch organization.

INITIAL RESPONSE ORGANIZATION - Initial Response resources are managed by the IC who will handle all Command and General Staff responsibilities. A UC is established. See Page 19-6 for an example of an oil spill initial response organization.

REINFORCED RESPONSE ORGANIZATION - The UC has established a Protection Group and a Recovery Group to manage on-water activities and a shoreline division to manage land-based resources. An SOFR and IO have been assigned. See Page 19-7 for an example of a reinforced response.

MULTI-DIVISION/GROUP ORGANIZATION - The UC has assigned all Command Staff positions and established a number of Divisions and Groups as well as an OSC and PSC. Some Logistic Units are established. See Page 19-8 for an example of a multi-division/group organization.

MULTI-BRANCH ORGANIZATION - The IC has established all Command and General Staff positions and has established four branches. See Page 19-9 for an example of an oil spill multi-branch organization.

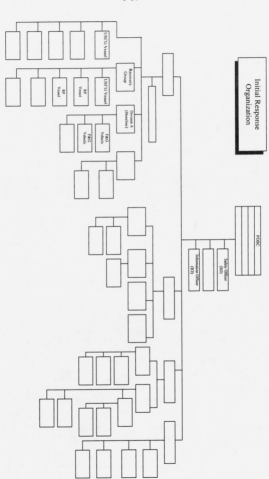

Initial Response Organization

FOSC

Information Officer (IO)

Safety Officer (SO)

Recovery Group

USCG Vessel

RP Vessel

RP Vessel

USCG Vessel

Division A (Shoreline)

F&G Vehicle

F&G Vehicle

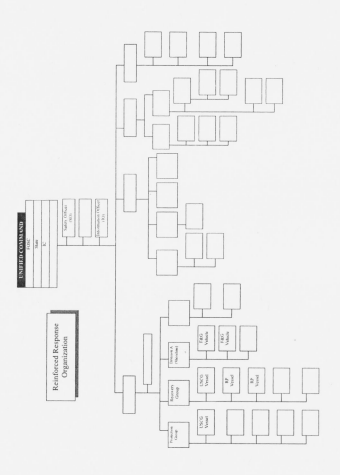

OIL SPILL

OIL SPILL

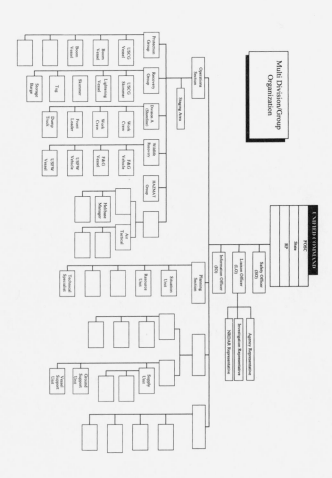

Multi Division/Group
Organization

UNIFIED COMMAND
FOSC
State
RP

Safety Officer (SO)
Liaison Officer (LO)
Information Officer (IO)

Agency Representative
Investigation Representative
NRDAR Representative

Operations Section

Staging Area

Protection Group
- USCG Vessel
- Boom Vessel

Recovery Group
- USCG Skimmer
- Lightering Vessel
- Skimmer
- Tug
- Storage Barge

Division A (Shoreline)
- Work Crew
- Front Loader
- Dump Truck

Wildlife Recovery
- F&G Vehicle
- F&G Vessel
- USFW Vehicle
- USFW Vessel

HAZMAT Group

Air Tactical
- Helibase Manager

Planning Section

Situation Unit

Resource Unit

Technical Specialist

Supply Unit

Ground Support Unit

Vessel Support Unit

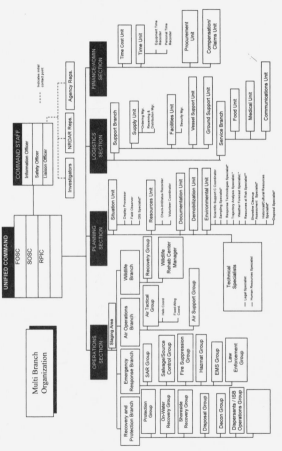

OIL SPILL SPECIFIC ICS POSITIONS AND TASK DESCRIPTIONS

INCIDENT COMMANDER – The IC for oil discharges will, whenever possible and practical, be organized under the UC Structure that includes, but is not limited to:

- The pre-designated FOSC
- The pre-designated State On-Scene Incident Commander (SOSC)
- The representative of the RP IC

The UC is responsible for the overall management of the incident. The UC directs incident activities including the development and implementation of strategic decisions and approves the ordering and releasing of resources. The UC may assign a Deputy IC to assist in carrying out IC responsibilities. IC tasks specific to oil spill events are:

a. Review IC Responsibilities in Chapter 6.
b. Review IC Job Aid.
c. Be cognizant of the primary objectives for oil spill response activities.
- Ensure the safety of citizens and response personnel.
- Control the source of the spill.
- Manage a coordinated response effort.
- Maximize protection of environmentally sensitive areas.
- Contain and recover spilled material.
- Recover and rehabilitate injured wildlife.
- Remove oil from impacted areas.
- Minimize economic impacts.
- Keep stakeholders informed of response activities.
- Keep the public informed of response

activities.

- Ensure that the source of a discharge is designated and that the RP advertises procedures by which claims may be presented or that the National Pollution Fund Center (NPFC) assumes this role.
- Inform the NPFC regarding the source of the discharge. NPFC will issue the required Notice of Designation.
- Refer all removal and damage claims to the RP or, if no identifiable RP, to the NPFC Claims Adjudication division.

FINANCE/ADMINISTRATION SECTION CHIEF – Refer to Page 10-2 for the Finance/Administration Section Chief position responsibilities. In addition, consult the References (d) and (e) for guidance on oil spill financial issues.

NRDAR REPRESENTATIVE - The Natural Resource Damage Assessment and Restoration (NRDAR) Representatives are responsible for coordinating NRDAR needs and activities of the trustee team. NRDAR activities generally do not occur within the structure, processes, and control of the ICS. However, particularly in the early phases of a spill response, many NRDAR activities overlap with the environmental assessment performed for the sake of spill response. Therefore, NRDAR Representatives should remain coordinated with the spill response organization through the LO, and they may need to work directly with the UC, Planning Section, Operations Section, and the NOAA SSC to resolve any problems or address areas of overlap. This includes close coordination with the LO for obtaining timely information on the spill and injuries to natural resources.

While NRDAR resource requirements and costs may fall outside the responsibility of the Logistics and Finance/Administrative Sections, coordination is important. The NRDAR Representative will coordinate NRDAR or injury determination activities.

    a. Review Common Responsibilities in Chapter 2.

    b. Review Agency Representative Responsibilities in Chapter 6.

    c. Attend appropriate meetings to facilitate communication between NRDAR Team and IC/UC.

    d. Provide status reports.

    e. Coordinate with the LO, or the UC in the absence of an LO, to assure that NRDAR field activities do not conflict with response activities and to request logistical support for NRDAR field activities.

    f. Seek the FOSC's cooperation in acquiring response-related samples or results of sample analysis applicable to NRDAR; (e.g., spilled petroleum product from source and/or oil from contaminated wildlife).

    g. Support the UCs information needs through the IO.

    h. Interact with appropriate units to collect information requested by the NRDAR Team.

    i. Obtain necessary safety clearances for access to sampling sites.

    j. Coordinate with other organizations to identify personnel available for NRDAR.

AIR TACTICAL GROUP SUPERVISOR - Air Tactical Group Supervisor tasks specific to oil spill events are: The coordination and scheduling of aircraft operations intended to locate, observe, track, surveil, support dispersant applications, or to be used for other deliverable response application techniques, or report on the incident situation when fixed and/or rotary-wing aircraft are airborne at an incident. These coordination activities are normally performed by the Air Tactical Group Supervisor while airborne.

   a. Review Air Tactical Group Supervisor Responsibilities in Chapter 7.

   b. Obtain a briefing from the Air Operations Branch Director or the OPS.

   c. Coordinate dispersant, in-situ burning, and bioremediation application through the Air Operations Branch Director.

   d. Coordinate air surveillance mission scheduling and observer assignments with the SUL.

   e. Identify remote sensing technology that may enhance surveillance capabilities.

   f. Coordinate air surveillance observations and provide reports by the most direct methods available.

   g. Report on air surveillance and operations activities to the Air Operations Branch Director.

   h. Coordinate application-monitoring requirements with the Helicopter and Fixed-Wing Coordinators and the Situation Unit.

   i. Report on air application activities to the Air Operation Branch Director.

HELICOPTER COORDINATOR - Helicopter Coordinator tasks specific to oil spill events are: The coordination and scheduling of helicopter operations intended to locate, observe, track, surveil, or report on the incident situation. The Helicopter Coordinator coordinates the application of dispersants, in-situ burning agents and bioremediation agents.

AIR TANKER/FIXED-WING COORDINATOR – The Air Tanker/Fixed-Wing Coordinator tasks specific to oil spill events are: The scheduling of fixed wing operations

19-13

intended to locate, observe. track, surveil, or report on the incident situation. The Air Tanker/Fixed-Wing Coordinator coordinates the aerial application of dispersants, in-situ burning agents and bioremediation agents.

RECOVERY AND PROTECTION BRANCH DIRECTOR - The Recovery and Protection Branch Director is responsible for overseeing and implementing the protection, containment and cleanup activities established in the IAP.
   a. Review Branch Director responsibilities in Chapter 7.

PROTECTION GROUP SUPERVISOR - The Protection Group Supervisor is responsible for the deployment of containment, diversion, and adsorbent/absorbent materials in designated locations. Depending on the size of the incident, the Protection Group may be further divided into Teams, Task Forces and Single Resources.
   a. Review Division/Group Supervisor responsibilities in Chapter 7.
   b. Implement Protection Strategies in the IAP.
   c. Direct, coordinate, and assess the effectiveness of protective actions.
   d. Modify protective actions, as needed.
   e. Maintain Unit/Activity Log (ICS Form 214).

ON WATER RECOVERY GROUP SUPERVISOR - The On Water Recovery Group Supervisor is responsible for managing on water recovery operations in compliance with the IAP. The Group may be further divided into Teams, Task Forces and Single Resources.
   a. Review Division/Group Supervisor responsibilities in Chapter 7.
   b. Implement Recovery Strategies in the IAP.
   c. Direct, coordinate, and assess the effectiveness

19-14

of on water recovery actions.
d. Modify recovery actions as needed.
e. Maintain Unit Log (ICS 214-CG).

DISPERSANT OPERATIONS GROUP SUPERVISOR -
The Dispersants Operations Group Supervisor is responsible for coordinating all aspects of a dispersant operation. For aerial applications, the Group works closely with the Air Tactical Group Supervisor.
a. Review Division/Group Supervisor responsibilities in Chapter 7.
b. Determine resource needs.
c. Assist the Planning Section in the development of dispersant operations and monitoring plans.
d. Implement approved dispersant operations and monitoring plans.
e. Manage dedicated dispersant resources and coordinate required monitoring.
f. Coordinate required monitoring.
g. Maintain Unit (ICS 214-CG).

IN-SITU BURN OPERATIONS GROUP SUPERVISOR
The In-Situ Burn Operations Group Supervisor is responsible for coordinating all aspects of an in-situ burn operation. For aerial ignition, the Group works closely with the Air Tactical Group Supervisor.
a. Review Division/Group Supervisor responsibilities in Chapter 7.
b. Determine resource needs.
c. Assist the Planning Section in the development of in-situ burn operations and monitoring plans.
d. Implement approved in-situ burn operations and monitoring plans.
e. Manage dedicated in-situ burning resources.
f. Coordinate required monitoring.
g. Maintain Unit Log (ICS 214-CG).

SHORESIDE RECOVERY GROUP SUPERVISOR -
The Shoreside Recovery Group Supervisor is
responsible for managing shoreside cleanup operations
in compliance with the IAP. The Group may be further
divided into Strike Teams, Task Forces, and Single
Resources.
  a. Review Division/Group Supervisor responsibilities
     in Chapter 7.
  b. Implement Recovery Strategies in the IAP.
  c. Direct, coordinate, and assess effectiveness of
     shoreside recovery actions.
  d. Modify protective actions, as needed.
  e. Maintain Unit Log (ICS 214-CG).

DISPOSAL GROUP SUPERVISOR - The Disposal
Group Supervisor is responsible for coordinating the on-
site activities of personnel engaged in collecting,
storing, transporting, and disposing of waste materials.
Depending on the size and location of the spill, the
Disposal Group may be further divided into Teams,
Task Forces, and Single Resources.
  a. Review Division/Group Supervisor responsibilities
     in Chapter 7.
  b. Implement the Disposal Portion of the IAP.
  c. Ensure compliance with all hazardous waste laws
     and regulations.
  d. Maintain accurate records of recovered material.
  e. Maintain Unit Log (ICS 214-CG).

DECONTAMINATION GROUP SUPERVISOR - The
Decontamination Group Supervisor is responsible for
decontamination of personnel and response equipment
in compliance with approved statutes.
  a. Review Division/Group Supervisor responsibilities
     in Chapter 7.
  b. Implement Decontamination Plan.
  c. Determine resource needs.

   d.   Direct and coordinate decontamination activities.
   e.   Brief Site SOFR on conditions.
   f.   Maintain Unit Log (ICS 214-CG).

EMERGENCY RESPONSE BRANCH DIRECTOR -
The Emergency Response Branch Director is primarily
responsible for overseeing and implementing
emergency measures to protect life, mitigate further
damage to the environment, and stabilize the situation.
   a.   Review Branch Director responsibilities
        in Chapter 7.

**SALVAGE/SOURCE CONTROL GROUP
SUPERVISOR** - Under the direction of the Emergency
Response Branch Director, the Salvage/Source Control
Group Supervisor is responsible for coordinating and
directing all salvage/source control activities related to
the incident.
   a.   Review Division/Group Supervisor responsibilities
        in Chapter 7.
   b.   Coordinate the development of Salvage/Source
        Control Plan.
   c.   Determine Salvage/Source Control resource
        needs.
   d.   Direct and coordinate implementation of the
        Salvage/Source Control Plan.
   e.   Manage dedicated salvage/Source Control
        resources.
   f.   Maintain Unit Log (ICS 214-CG).

WILDLIFE BRANCH DIRECTOR - The Wildlife Branch
Director is responsible for minimizing wildlife injuries
during spill responses; coordinating early aerial and
ground reconnaissance of the wildlife at the spill site
and reporting results to the SUL; advising on wildlife
protection strategies, including diversionary booming
placements, in-situ burning, and chemical

countermeasures; removing of oiled carcasses, employing wildlife hazing measures as authorized in the IAP; and recovering and rehabilitating impacted wildlife. A central Wildlife Processing Center should be identified and maintained for, evidence tagging, transportation, veterinary services, treatment and rehabilitation storage, and other support needs. The activities of private wildlife care groups, including those employed by the RP, will be overseen and coordinated by the Wildlife Branch Director.

    a.   Review Branch Director responsibilities in Chapter 7.

    b.   Develop the Wildlife Branch portion of the IAP.

    c.   Supervise Wildlife Branch operations.

    d.   Determine resource needs.

    e.   Review the suggested list of resources to be released and initiate recommendation for release of resources.

    f.   Assemble and disassemble teams/task forces assigned to the Wildlife Branch.

    g.   Report information about special activities, events, and occurrences to the OPS.

    h.   Assist the Volunteer Coordinator in determining training needs of wildlife recovery volunteers.

    i.   Maintain Unit Log (ICS 214-CG)

WILDLIFE RECOVERY GROUP SUPERVISOR - The Wildlife Recovery Group Supervisor is responsible for coordinating the search for collection and field tagging of dead and live impacted wildlife and transporting them to the processing center(s). This group should coordinate with the Planning Situation Unit in conducting aerial and group surveys of wildlife population in the vicinity of the spill. They should also deploy acoustic and visual wildlife hazing equipment, as needed.

    a.   Review Division/Group Supervisor responsibilities

19-18

in Chapter 7.
b. Determine resource needs.
c. Establish and implement protocols for collection and logging of impacted wildlife.
d. Coordinate transportation of wildlife to processing stations(s).
e. Maintain Unit Log (ICS 214-CG).

WILDLIFE REHABILITATION CENTER MANAGER - The Wildlife Rehabilitation Center Manager is responsible for the oversight of facility operations, including: receiving oiled wildlife at the processing center, recording essential information, collecting necessary samples, and conducting triage, stabilization, treatment, transport and rehabilitation of oiled wildlife. The Wildlife Rehabilitation Center Manager is responsible for assuring appropriate transportation to appropriate treatment centers for oiled animals requiring extended care and treatment.
a. Review Common Responsibilities in Chapter 2.
b. Determine resource needs and establish a processing station for impacted wildlife.
c. Process impacted wildlife and maintain logs.
d. Collect numbers/types/status of impacted wildlife and brief the Wildlife Branch Operations Director.
e. Coordinate the transport of wildlife to other facilities.
f. Coordinate release of recovered wildlife.
g. Implement Incident Demobilization Plan.
h. Maintain Unit Log (ICS 214-CG).

SCIENTIFIC SUPPORT COORDINATOR - The Scientific Support Coordinator (SSC) is a technical specialist and is defined in the NCP as the principal advisor to the FOSC for scientific issues. The SSC is responsible for providing expertise on chemical hazards, field observations, trajectory analysis, resources at risk, environmental tradeoffs of countermeasures and cleanup methods, and information management. The SSC is also charged with gaining consensus on scientific issues affecting the response, but also ensuring that differing opinions within the scientific community are communicated to the incident command. Additionally, the SSC is responsible for providing data on weather, tides, currents, and other applicable environmental conditions. The SSC can serve as the Environmental Unit Leader.

a. Review Common Responsibilities in Chapter 2.
b. Review Technical Specialist Job Aid.
c. Attend planning meetings.
d. Determine resource needs.
e. Provide overflight maps and trajectory analysis, including the actual location of oil, to the Situation Unit.
f. Provide weather, tidal and current information.
g. Obtain consensus on scientific issues affecting the response.
h. In conjunction with Natural Resource Trustee Representatives and the FOSC's Historical/Cultural Resources Specialist, develop a prioritized list of resources at risk, including threatened and endangered species.
i. Provide information on chemical hazards.
j. Evaluate environmental tradeoffs of countermeasures and cleanup methods, and response endpoints.
k. Maintain Unit Log (ICS 214-CG)

SAMPLING TECHNICIAL SPECIALIST - The Sampling Technical Specialist is responsible for providing a sampling plan for the coordinated collection, documentation, storage, transportation, and submittal to appropriate laboratories for analysis or storage.

a. Review Common Responsibilities in Chapter 2.

19-20

OIL SPILL   **OIL SPILL**

b. Review Technical Specialist Job Aid.
c. Determine resource needs.
d. Participate in planning meetings as required.
e. Identify and alert appropriate laboratories.
f. Meet with team to develop an initial sampling plan and strategy, and review sampling and labeling procedures.
g. Set up site map to monitor the location of samples collected and coordinate with GIS staff. Coordinate sampling activities with the NRDAR Representative, Investigation Team, and legal advisors.
h. Provide status reports to appropriate requesters.
i. Maintain Unit Log (ICS 214-CG).

RESPONSE TECHNOLOGIES SPECIALIST - The Response Technologies Specialist is responsible for evaluating the opportunities to use various response technologies, including mechanical containment and recovery, dispersant or other chemical countermeasures, in-situ burning, and bioremediation. The specialist will conduct the consultation and planning required by deploying a specific response technology, and by articulating the environmental tradeoffs of using or not using a specific response technique.
a. Review Common Responsibilities in Chapter 2.
b. Review Technical Specialist Job Aid.
c. Participate in planning meetings, as required.
d. Determine resource needs.
e. Gather data pertaining to the spill, including spill location, type and amount of petroleum spilled, physical and chemical properties, weather and sea conditions, and resources at risk.
f. Identify the available response technologies (RT) that may be effective on the specific spilled petroleum.
g. Make initial notification to all agencies that have

19-21

authority over the use of RT.
h. Keep the PSC advised of RT issues.
i. Provide status reports to appropriate requesters.
j. Establish communications with the RRT to coordinate RT activities.
k. Maintain Unit Log (ICS 214-CG).

TRAJECTORY ANALYSIS TECHNICAL SPECIALIST -
The Trajectory Analysis Technical Specialist is responsible for providing to the UC, projections and estimates of the movement and behavior of the spill. The specialist will combine visual observations, remote sensing information, and computer modeling, as well as observed and predicted tidal, current, and weather data to form these analyses.

Additionally, the specialist is responsible for interfacing with local experts (weather service, academia, researchers, etc.) in formulating these analyses. Trajectory maps, over-flight maps, tides and current data, and weather forecasts will be supplied by the specialist to the Situation Unit for dissemination throughout the ICP.
a. Review Common Responsibilities in Chapter 2.
b. Review Technical Specialist Job Aid.
c. Schedule and conduct spill observations/over-flights, as needed.
d. Gather pertinent information on tides, currents and weather from all available sources.
e. Provide a trajectory and over-flight maps, weather forecasts, and tidal and current information.
f. Provide briefing on observations and analyses to the proper personnel.
g. Demobilize in accordance with the Incident Demobilization Plan.
h. Maintain Unit Log (ICS 214-CG).

19-22

WEATHER FORECAST TECHNICAL SPECIALIST -
The Weather Forecast Technical Specialist is responsible for acquiring and reporting incident-specific weather forecasts. The specialist will interpret and analyze data from NOAA's National Weather Service and other sources. This person will be available to answer specific weather related response questions and coordinate with the Scientific Support Coordinator and Trajectory Analysis Specialist as needed. The specialist will provide weather forecasts to the Situation Unit for dissemination throughout the ICP.
  a. Review Common Responsibilities in Chapter 2.
  b. Gather pertinent weather information from all appropriate sources.
  c. Provide incident-specific weather forecasts on an assigned schedule.
  d. Provide briefings on weather observations and forecasts to the proper personnel.
  e. Maintain Unit Log (ICS 214-CG).

RESOURCES AT RISK (RAR) TECHNICAL SPECIALIST -
The Resources at Risk (RAR) Technical Specialist is responsible for the identification of resources thought to be at risk from exposure to the spilled oil through the analysis of known and anticipated oil movement, and the location of natural, economic resources, and historic properties. The RAR Technical Specialist considers the relative importance of the resources and the relative risk to develop a priority list for protection.
  a. Review Common Responsibilities in Chapter 2.
  b. Review Technical Specialist Job Aid.
  c. Participate in planning meetings as required.
  d. Determine resource needs.
  e. Obtain current and forecasted status information from the Situation Unit.

19-23

    f.   Following consultation with Natural Resource Trustee Representatives, identify natural RAR, including threatened and endangered species, and their critical habitat.

    g.   Following consultation with the FOSC's Historical/Cultural Resources Specialist, identify historic properties at risk.

    h.   Identify socio-economic resources at risk.

    i.   In consultation with Natural Resource Trustee Representatives, Land Management Agency Representatives, and the FOSC's Historical/Cultural Resources Specialist, develop a prioritized list of the resources at risk for use by the Planning Section.

    j.   Provide status reports to appropriate requesters.

    k.   Maintain Unit Log (ICS 214-CG).

SHORELINE CLEANUP ASSESSMENT TECHNICAL SPECIALIST The Shoreline Cleanup Assessment Technical Specialist is responsible for providing appropriate cleanup recommendations as to the types of the various shorelines and the degree to which they have been impacted. This technical specialist will recommend the need for, and the numbers of, Shoreline Cleanup Assessment Teams (SCATs) and will be responsible for making cleanup recommendations to the Environmental Unit Leader. Additionally, this specialist will recommend cleanup endpoints that address the question of "**How clean is clean?**"

    a.   Review Common Responsibilities in Chapter 2.

    b.   Review Technical Specialist Job Aid.

    c.   Obtain a briefing and special instructions from the Environmental Unit Leader.

    d.   Participate in Planning Section meetings.

    e.   Recommend the need for and number of SCATs.

    f.   Describe shoreline types and oiling conditions.

    g.   Identify sensitive resources (ecological,

recreational, historical properties, economic).
h. Recommend the need for cleanup. In consultation with Natural Resource Trustee Representatives, Land Management Agency Representatives, and the FOSC's Historical/Cultural Resources Specialist.
i. Recommend cleanup priorities. In consultation with Natural Resource Trustee Representatives, Land Management Agency Representatives, and the FOSC's Historical/Cultural Resources Specialist.
j. Monitor cleanup effectiveness.
k. Recommend shoreline cleanup methods and endpoints
l. Maintain Unit Log (ICS 214-CG).

HISTORICAL/CULTURAL RESOURCES TECHNICAL SPECIALIST - The Historical/Cultural Resources Technical Specialist is responsible for identifying and resolving issues related to any historical or cultural sites that are threatened or impacted during an incident. The Specialist must understand and be able to implement a "Programmatic Agreement on Protection of Historic Properties" (Consult NRT's document "Programmatic Agreement on the Protection of Historic Properties During Emergency Response under the NCP" for guidance) as well as consulting with State Historic Preservation Officers (SHPO), land management agencies, appropriate native tribes and organizations, and other concerned parties. The technical specialist must identify historical/cultural sites and develop strategies for protection and cleanup of those sites in order to minimize damage.
a. Review Common Responsibilities in Chapter 2.
b. Review Agency Representative Responsibilities in Chapter 6.
c. Review Technical Specialist Job Aid.

19-25

    d. Implement the Programmatic Agreement (PA) for the FOSC.

    e. If a PA is not used, coordinate Section 106 consultations with the SHPO.

    f. Consult and reach consensus with the concerned parties on affected historical/cultural sites.

    g. Identify and prioritize threatened or impacted historical/cultural sites.

    h. Develop response strategies to protect historical/cultural sites.

    i. Participate in the testing and evaluation of cleanup techniques used on historical/cultural sites.

    j. Ensure compliance with applicable Federal/State regulations.

    k. Maintain Unit Log (ICS 214-CG).

DISPOSAL (WASTE MANAGEMENT) TECHNICAL SPECIALIST - The Disposal (Waste Management) Technical Specialist is responsible for providing the OSC with a Disposal Plan that details the collection, sampling, monitoring, temporary storage, transportation, recycling, and disposal of all anticipated response wastes.

    a. Review Common Responsibilities in Chapter 2.

    b. Review Technical Specialist Job Aid.

    c. Determine resource needs.

    d. Participate in planning meetings as required.

    e. Develop a Pre-Cleanup Plan and monitor pre-cleanup operations, if appropriate.

    f. Develop a detailed Waste Management Plan.

    g. Calculate and verify the volume of petroleum recovered, including petroleum collected with sediment/sand, etc.

    h. Provide status reports to appropriate requesters.

    i. Maintain Unit Log (ICS 214-CG).

CHAPTER 20

HAZARDOUS SUBSTANCE
(Chemical, Biological, Radiological, and Nuclear)

CHAPTER 20

HAZARDOUS SUBSTANCE
(Chemical, Biological, Radiological, and Nuclear)

References:
  (a) National Response Plan (NRP)
  (b) National Incident Management System (NIMS)
  (c) National Contingency Plan (NCP)
  (d) Technical Specialist Job Aid

INTRODUCTION

There are numerous scenarios that provide an opportunity for the Coast Guard to become involved in Hazardous Substance/Material (CBRN- Chemical, Biological, Radiological, Nuclear) releases. The Coast Guard is a regulatory agency for industries involved in the transport of hazardous substances, routinely supports other agencies in their response to hazardous substance releases, and may become involved in hazardous substance releases when responding or supporting responses to other incidents such as terrorist actions, oil spills from refrigerated cargo ships, accidents at non-transportation related facilities that may be located within a COTP Zone, etc. It is impossible to address all possible ICS organizations that may result from the above scenarios. Therefore, this chapter will review two possible scenarios involving hazardous substances/materials. One will be a land based facility type event, and the second a will be marine type incident in an offshore area. Both will show the modular development of the ICS organization.

It is important to note that the majority of hazardous substance releases, like oil spills, are small events that will not and should not result in a response beyond that

20-2

of an initial or reinforced response organization. It should also be noted that the capabilities in various COTP zones throughout the country vary greatly. The COTP must have knowledge of the local government response capability and be familiar with their ICs as this will affect the degree of leadership and control that the Coast Guard will be expected to take in hazardous substance/material events. In areas where the state and local government have a strong hazardous substance/materials response program, the Coast Guard may be primarily in a support role during the emergency phases. In areas where there is no hazardous substance capability, the Coast Guard may be expected to take a much stronger leadership role.

In this regard, there may also be reasons to expand the UC beyond the FOSC, SOSC, and Responsible Party IC (RPIC) participation that has become the standard for oil spill response. The UC represented in this chapter reflects the possible levels of participation that may be seen in some locations and situations for hazardous substance incidents. Annual pre-incident planning meetings of all possible stakeholders are essential and highly recommended for determining the response capabilities and personalities that may be involved in the real event for a specific local area or region. These annual meetings will assist the FOSC in determining what level of UC participation will be required for his/her area.

There are different definitions used for hazardous response throughout the transportation, response and regulatory communities. Hazardous substances are referred to as hazardous materials, noxious substances, chemicals, biological, radiological, nuclear, CBRN, and other names. In this section, you will find "hazardous substances" referred to as hazardous substance/material.

This is in consideration of the fact that in laws that are the basis for Coast Guard response authority (OPA-90, CERCLA, RCRA) the term hazardous substance is used, however, fire and police departments nationwide refer to chemical response activity as hazardous materials response. Since most hazardous substance responses will include City, County, Regional, and State Fire and Law Enforcement Agencies, the ICS organizations in this section will include both terms.

The organizations have been modified in this section to reflect that under OPA 90 regulations, the responsible party (RP) who has had the release is mandated to follow an approved Facility Response Plan (FRP) or Vessel Response Plan (VRP), to provide a spill management team for managing the release, and to become a member of the UC.

Response to a biological incident in the coastal zone can range from the illegal disposal of medical waste to the intentional release of a disease-causing organism. Initial response actions to a biological incident will depend on the type of incident and the cause/or suspected cause of the incident (i.e. terrorist act).

The Coast Guard Incident Commander's response to biological incidents most likely will involve the use of both the Captain of the Port and Federal On-scene Coordinator (FOSC) authorities. The FOSC role is limited to disease causing agents that exist outside a host for a period of time and which can be physically removed from the environment.

If the biological incident is suspected or confirmed to be the result of a terrorist act, response to the incident should be initiated using this Chapter, the Terrorism Chapter, the National Response Plan, and the Area Maritime Security Plan.

A radiological incident involves the release or potential release of radioactive material that poses an actual or perceived hazard to public safety, national security and/or the environment.

The U.S. Coast Guard's jurisdiction as the Coordinating Agency for a radiological incident is limited in both geographic area and authority. In radiological incidents where the Coast Guard has jurisdiction and there is no involvement of terrorism the Coast Guard Incident Commander responds under the NCP. For any radiological incidents where terrorism is involved, the Department of Energy is the Coordinating Agency responding under the NRP and the Coast Guard is a cooperating agency. The National Response Plan limits the Coast Guard's Coordinating Agency role for radiological incidents to "*certain areas of the coastal zone.*" In addition to geographic limitations, the scope of the Coast Guard's jurisdiction as the Coordinating Agency is limited to those radiological incidents that do not involve a terrorist act.

The role of Coordinating Agency for radiological incidents in the maritime environment can reside with several different federal agencies depending on geographic location, accountability for the radiological source, and the suspected or actual involvement of terrorism.

For any terrorist event involving non-Department of Defense or non-Nuclear Regulatory Committee (NRC) radioactive material, the Department of Energy (DOE) will assume the role of Coordinating Agency to address the radiological aspects of the response. Please see the NRP for more information.

The Hazardous Substance/Materials organization module is designed to provide an organization structure that will provide necessary supervision and control for the essential functions required at virtually all Hazardous Substance/Materials incidents. This is based on the premise that controlling the tactical operations of companies and movement of personnel and equipment will provide a greater degree of safety and also reduce the probability of spreading of contaminants. The Hazardous Substance/Materials Group Supervisor will direct the primary functions, and all resources that have a direct involvement with hazardous materials will be supervised by one of the functional leaders, the Hazardous Substances/Materials Group Supervisor, or when activated the Hazardous Substances/Materials Branch Director.

Since the Logistics Section and Finance Sections, if formed during a hazardous substance response, will reflect the same functional requirements as in the generic ICS organization, they have not been included in the organizational charts for this chapter.

UNIFIED COMMAND

A hazardous substances/materials release may bring together a greater number and a wider variety of agencies than any other single incident the Coast Guard may face. It is assumed that all hazardous materials incidents will be managed under UC principles because in virtually all cases, fire, law enforcement, and public health agencies will have some statutory functional responsibility for IC and Control and mitigation.

Depending on incident factors, several other agencies will respond to a hazardous materials incident. The best method of ensuring effective information flow and coordination between the responding agencies at the scene of a multi-agency incident is to establish an ICP and the use of a UC. Each key response agency should provide a representative to remain at the ICP who will have authority to speak for and commit agency resources. The Assisting Agencies Section of this document lists some of the typical functional responsibilities of law enforcement and health agencies.

HAZARDOUS SUBSTANCE SCENARIO AND MODULAR ORGANIZATION DEVELOPEMENT

MODULAR DEVELOPMENT FOR A LAND BASED TYPE EVENT - A series of examples of modular development are included to illustrate one method of expanding the incident organization.

INITIAL RESPONSE ORGANIZATION (LAND BASED TYPE EVENT) - The ICs will handle all Command and General Staff responsibilities and manage initial response resources. See Page 20-9 for an example of an Initial Response Organization.

REINFORCED RESPONSE ORGANIZATION (LAND BASED TYPE EVENT) - The two IC's have met and have established a UC. They have established a Hazardous Materials Group to manage all activities around the Control Zones and have organized Law Enforcement Units into a Task Force to isolate the Operational Area. The IC's have decided to establish a Planning Section, a Staging Area and a SO. See Page 20-10 for an example of a Reinforced Response Organization.

MULTI-DIVISION/GROUP ORGANIZATION (LAND BASED TYPE EVENT) - The UC has activated most Command and General Staff positions and has established a combination of Divisions and Groups. See Page 20-11 for an example of a Multi-Division/Group Organization

MULTI BRANCH ORGANIZATION FOR A LAND BASED TYPE EVENT - The UC has activated all Command and General Staff positions and has established four branches in the OPS. See Page 20-12 for an example of a Multi-Branch Organization.

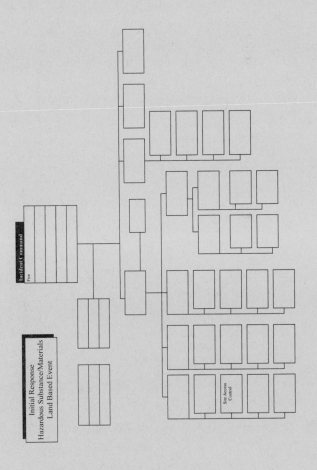

HAZARDOUS SUBSTANCE   HAZARDOUS SUBSTANCE

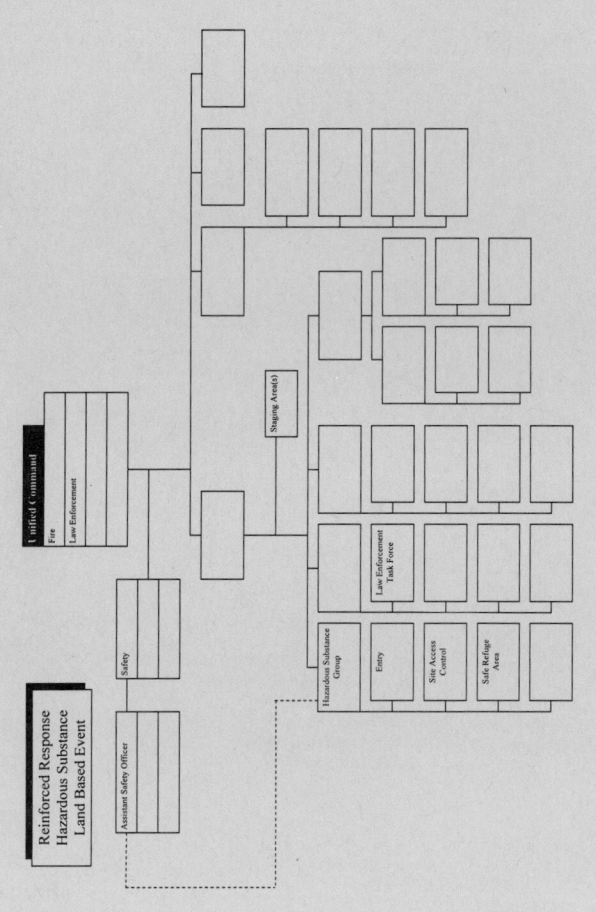

20-10

HAZARDOUS SUBSTANCE   HAZARDOUS SUBSTANCE

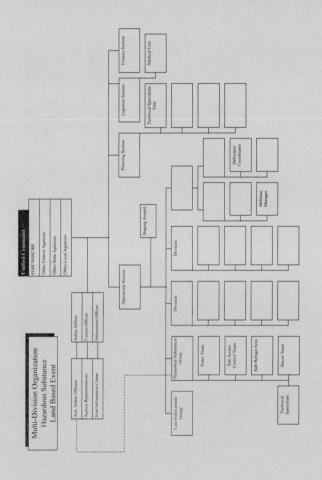

Multi-Division Organization
Hazardous Substance
Land Based Event

Unified Command
FOSC/SOSC/RP
Other Federal Agencies
Other State Agencies
Other Local Agencies

Safety Officer
Liaison Officer
Information Officer

Asst Safety Officers
Agency Representatives
Joint Information Center

Operations Section
Planning Section
Logistics Section
Finance Section

Staging Area(s)

Technical Specialists Unit
Medical Unit

Law Enforcement Group
Hazardous Substances Group
Division
Division

Entry Team
Site Access Control Team
Safe Refuge Area
Decon Team

Helibase Manager
Helicopter Coordinator

Technical Specialists

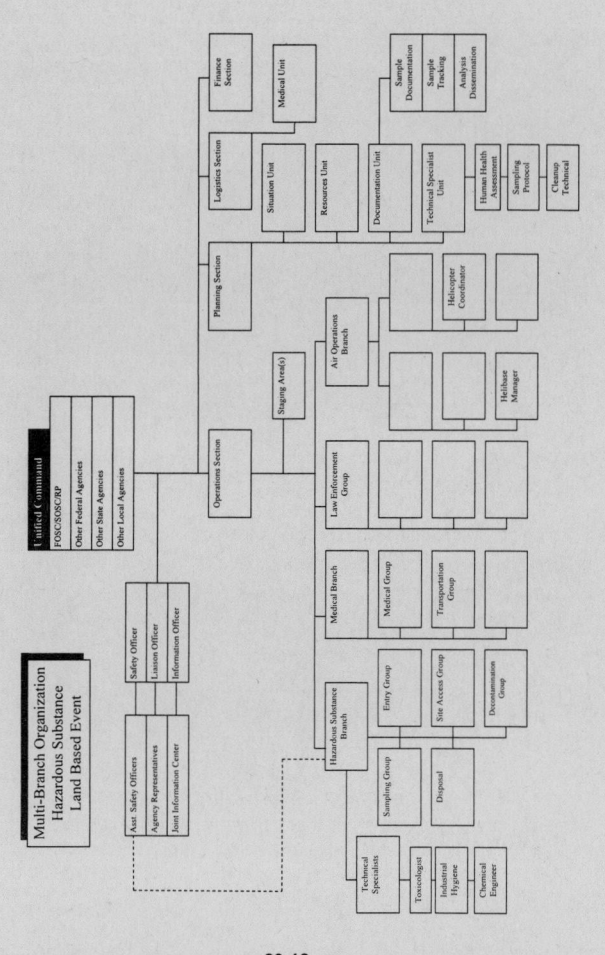

20-12

MODULAR DEVELOPMENT (MARINE TYPE EVENT)

INITIAL RESPONSE ORGANIZATION (MARINE TYPE EVENT) - A vessel offshore suffers a casualty that releases a hazardous substance. The initial IC will be the vessel's master, and the ship's crew will carry out initial response activities. The Coast Guard will be involved from a notification perspective and will begin assessment of the situation based on information from the master. See Page 20-14 for an example of an Initial Response Organization.

REINFORCED RESPONSE ORGANIZATION (MARINE TYPE EVENT) - The FOSC and the vessel's QI/owner representative have met and have established a UC. They have established two Hazardous Materials Groups to fully assess the situation and plan a response. See Page 20-15 for an example of a Reinforced Response Organization.

MULTI-DIVISION/GROUP ORGANIZATION (MARINE TYPE EVENT) - The UC has activated most Command and General Staff positions and has molded the RP and government resources into a combination of Groups tasked with assessing and responding to the incident. See Page 20-16 for an example of a Multi-Division/Group Organization.

MULTI BRANCH ORGANIZATION (MARINE TYPE EVENT) - The UC has activated all Command and General Staff positions and has established four branches within the OPS. Since the event may require action to bring the vessel into port for offloading, firefighting, or salvage and repair, the UC includes state and city representation. See Page 20-17 for an example of a Multi-Branch Organization.

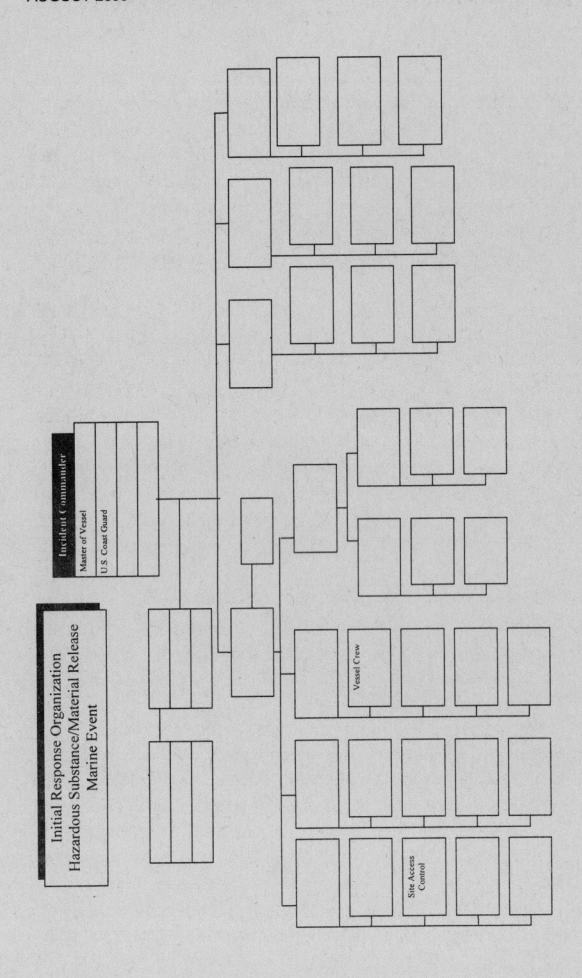

HAZARDOUS SUBSTANCE   **HAZARDOUS SUBSTANCE**

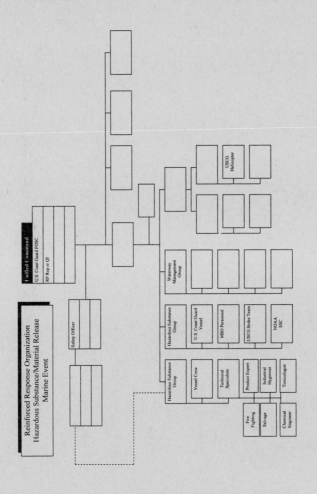

Reinforced Response Organization
Hazardous Substance/Material Release
Marine Event

Unified Command
U.S. Coast Guard FOSC
RP Rep or QI

Safety Officer

Waterway Management Group

USCG Helicopter

Hazardous Substance Group
U.S. Coast Guard Vessel
MSO Personnel
USCG Strike Team
NOAA SSC

Hazardous Substance Group
Vessel Crew
Technical Specialists
Product Expert
Industrial Hygienist
Toxicologist

Fire Fighting
Salvage
Chemical Engineer

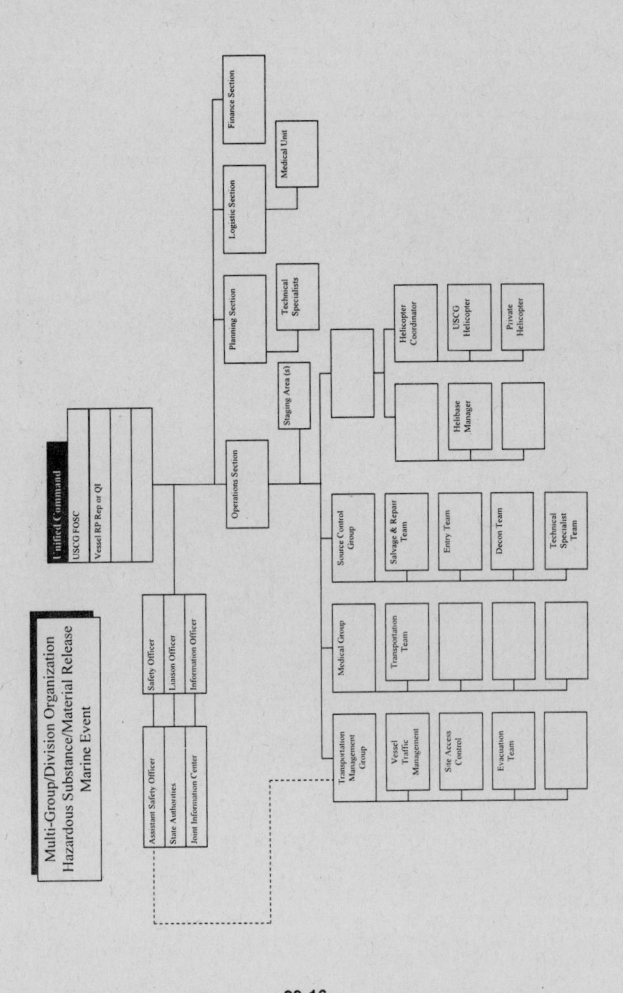

Multi-Group/Division Organization
Hazardous Substance/Material Release
Marine Event

Unified Command
USCG FOSC
Vessel RP Rep or QI

Safety Officer
Liaison Officer
Information Officer

Assistant Safety Officer
State Authorities
Joint Information Center

Operations Section
Planning Section
Logistic Section
Finance Section

Technical Specialists
Medical Unit

Staging Area (s)

Source Control Group
Salvage & Repair Team
Entry Team
Decon Team
Technical Specialist Team

Medical Group
Transportation Team

Transportation Management Group
Vessel Traffic Management
Site Access Control
Evacuation Team

Helicopter Coordinator
USCG Helicopter
Private Helicopter

Helibase Manager

20-16

HAZARDOUS SUBSTANCE   **HAZARDOUS SUBSTANCE**

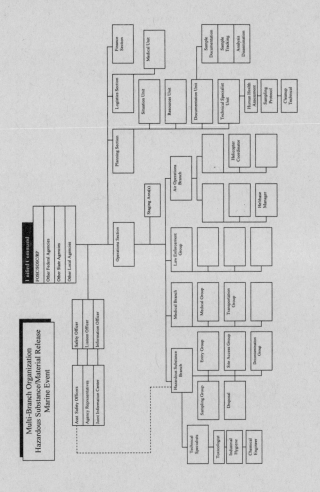

HAZARDOUS SUBSTANCE   HAZARDOUS SUBSTANCE

HAZARDOUS SUBSTANCE/HAZMAT RELEASE SPECIFIC ICS POSITIONS AND TASK DESCRIPTIONS

Only those positions and tasks specific and unique to Hazardous Substance/Material Release response missions will be described in this section. Persons assigned to positions common and consistent with the NIIMS organization should refer to the position job aids and Chapter 5-11 of this IMH for their position/task description checklists.

INCIDENT COMMANDER and SAFETY OFFICER - In addition to the specific tasks assigned to the IC and SOFR on Page 6-2 and Page 6-6, respectively, the IC and SOFR for a hazardous substance incident will use the following guidance when preparing the Site Safety Plan:

a. Assign site safety responsibility.
b. Establish perimeter and restrict access.
c. Characterize site hazards:
   • Identity pollutant.
   • Obtain Material Safety Data Sheets.
   • Conduct air monitoring.
   • Identify physical and biological hazards i.e.: slips, trips, falls, confined spaces, noise, weather conditions, poisonous insects, reptiles, plants and biological waste.
d. Establish control zones:
   • Exclusion zone.
   • Contamination reduction zone.
   • Support zone.
e. Assess training requirements:
   • Check HAZWOPER cards.
   • Insure safety briefings.

   f.   Select personal protective equipment (PPE):
- Level A, B, C, or D.

   g. Establish decontamination stations.

   h. Establish Emergency Medical Plan:
- Locate and list: hospital, EMT(S) and first-aid stations.
- List emergency numbers: fire, police, and ambulance.

ASSISTANT SAFETY OFFICER – HAZARDOUS MATERIALS - The Assistant Safety Officer coordinates with the Hazardous Substance/Material Group Supervisor (or Hazardous Materials Branch Director, (if activated). The Assistant Safety Officer Hazardous Substance/Material coordinates safety related activities directly relating to the Hazardous Substance/Material Group operations as mandated by 29 CFR Part 1910.120 and applicable State and local laws. The person in this position advises the Hazardous Substance/Material Group Supervisor (or Hazardous Substance/Material Branch Director) on all aspects of health and safety and has the authority to stop or prevent unsafe acts. In a multi-activity incident the Assistant Safety Officer Hazardous Substance/Material does not act as the Safety Officer for the overall incident. Assistant Site Safety Officer-Hazardous Substance/Material tasks include:

   a. Review SOFR Responsibilities in Chapter 6.

   b. Obtain a briefing from the Hazardous Substance/Material Group Supervisor.

   c. Participate in the preparation and implementation of a Site Safety and Control Plan.

   d. Advise the Hazardous Substance/Material Group Supervisor (or Hazardous Substance/Material Branch Director) of deviations from the Site Safety and Control Plan (ICS Form 208-HM) or any dangerous situations.

   e. Alter, suspend, or terminate any activity that is judged to be unsafe.

   f. Ensure the protection of the Hazardous Substance/Material Group personnel from physical, environmental, and chemical hazards/exposures.

   g. Ensure the provision of required emergency medical services for assigned personnel and coordinate with the Medical Unit Leader.

   h. Ensure that medical related records for the Hazardous Substance/Material Group personnel are maintained.

   i. Maintain Unit Log (ICS 214-CG).

FINANCE/ADMINISTRATION SECTION CHIEF - Refer to Page 10-2 for the Finance/Administration Section Chief position responsibilities. In addition, consult the NPFC user reference Guides (TOPS) and the FFARM Field Guide for guidance on hazardous material financial issues.

HAZARDOUS SUBSTANCE/MATERIAL GROUP SUPERVISOR - The Hazardous Substance/Material Group Supervisor is responsible for the implementation of the phases of the IAP dealing with the Hazardous Material Group operations. The Hazardous Substance/Material Group Supervisor is responsible for the assignment of resources within the Hazardous Substance/Material Group, reporting on the progress of control operations and the status of resources within the Group. The Hazardous Substance/Material Group Supervisor directs the overall operations of the

Hazardous Substance/Materials Group; Additional tasks include:

   a. Review Division/Group Supervisor Responsibilities in Chapter 7.

   b. Ensure the development of Control Zones and Access Control Points and the placement of appropriate control lines.

   c. Evaluate and recommend public protection action options to the OSC or Branch Director (if activated).

   d. Ensure that current weather data and future weather predictions are obtained.

   e. Establish environmental monitoring of the hazard site for contaminants.

   f. Ensure that a Site Safety and Control Plan (ICS Form 208-HM) is developed and implemented.

   g. Conduct safety meetings with the Hazardous Substance/Material Group.

   h. Participate, when requested, in the development of the IAP.

   i. Ensure that recommended safe operational procedures are followed.

   j. Ensure that the proper Personal Protective Equipment is selected and used.

   k. Ensure that the appropriate agencies are notified through the Incident Commander.

   l. Maintain Unit/Activity Log (ICS Form 214).

ENTRY LEADER - Reports to the Hazardous Substance/Material Group Supervisor. The Entry Leader is responsible for the overall entry operations of assigned personnel within the Exclusion Zone; Additional tasks include:

   a. Review Unit Leader Responsibilities in Chapter 2.

   b. Supervise entry operations.

   c. Recommend actions to mitigate the situation within the Exclusion Zone.

d. Carry out actions, as directed by the Hazardous Substance/Material Group Supervisor.

e. Maintain communications and coordinate operations with the Decontamination Leader.

f. Maintain communications and coordinate operations with the Site Access Control Leader and the Safe Refuge Area Manager (if activated).

g. Maintain communications and coordinate operations with the Technical Specialist Hazardous Substance/Material Reference.

h. Maintain control of the movement of people and equipment within the Exclusion Zone, including contaminated victims.

i. Direct rescue operations, as needed, in the Exclusion Zone.

j. Maintain Unit Log (ICS 214-CG).

DECONTAMINATION GROUP SUPERVISOR - The Decontamination Group Supervisor is responsible for the operations of the decontamination element and for providing decontamination, as required by the ICP; Additional tasks include:.

a. Review Division/Group Supervisor Responsibilities in Chapter 7.

b. Establish the Contamination Reduction Corridor(s).

c. Identify contaminated people and equipment.

d. Supervise the operations of the decontamination element in the process of decontaminating people and equipment.

e. Maintain control of movement of people and equipment within the Contamination Reduction Zone.

f. Maintain communications and coordinate operations with the Entry Leader.

g. Maintain communications and coordinate operations with the Site Access Control Leader

20-22

and the Safe Refuge Area Manager (if activated).

h. Coordinate the transfer of contaminated patients requiring medical attention (after decontamination) to the Medical Group.

i. Coordinate handling, storage, and transfer of contaminants within the Contamination Reduction Zone.

j. Maintain Unit Log (ICS 214-CG).

SITE ACCESS CONTROL LEADER - The Site Access Control Leader is responsible for the control of the movement of all people and equipment through appropriate access routes at the hazard site and ensures that contaminants are controlled and records are maintained.

a. Review Unit Leader Responsibilities in Chapter 2.

b. Organize and supervise assigned personnel to control access to the hazard site.

c. Oversee the placement of the Exclusion Control Line and the Contamination Control Line.

c. Ensure that appropriate action is taken to prevent the spread of contamination.

d. Establish the Safe Refuge Area within the Contamination Reduction Zone. Appoint a Safe Refuge Area Manager (as needed).

e. Ensure that injured or exposed individuals are decontaminated prior to departure from the hazard site.

f. Track the movement of persons passing through the Contamination Control Line to ensure that long-term observations are provided.

g. Coordinate with the Medical Group for proper separation and tracking of potentially contaminated individuals needing medical attention.

h. Maintain observations of any changes in climatic conditions or other circumstances external to the

20-23

hazard site.
i.   Maintain communications and coordinate operations with the Entry Leader.
j.   Maintain communications and coordinate operations with the Decontamination Leader.
k.   Maintain Unit Log (ICS 214-CG).

SAFE REFUGE AREA MANAGER - The Safe Refuge Area Manager reports to the Site Access Control Leader and coordinates with the Decontamination Leader and the Entry Leader. The Safe Refuge Area Manager is responsible for evaluating and prioritizing victims for treatment, collecting information from the victims, and preventing the spread of contamination by these victims. If there is a need for the Safe Refuge Area Manager to enter the Contamination Reduction Zone in order to fulfill assigned responsibilities then the appropriate PPE shall be worn.
a.   Maintain Common Responsibilities in Chapter 2.
b.   Establish the Safe Refuge Area within the Contamination Reduction Zone adjacent to the Contamination Reduction Corridor and the Exclusion Control Line.
c.   Monitor the hazardous substance/materials release to ensure that the Safe Refuge Area is not subject to exposure.
d.   Assist the Site Access Control Leader by ensuring the victims are evaluated for contamination.
e.   Manage the Safe Refuge Area for the holding and evaluation of victims who may have information about the incident, or if they are suspected of having contamination.
f.   Maintain communications with the Entry Leader to coordinate the movement of victims from the Refuge Area(s) in the Exclusion Zone to the Safe Refuge Area.
g.   Maintain communications with the

Decontamination Leader to coordinate the movement of victims from the Safe Refuge Area into the Contamination Reduction Corridor, if needed.

h. Maintain Unit Log (ICS 214-CG).

SAMPLING GROUP SUPERVISOR - The Sampling Group is assigned to the Operations Section because of the immediate communication and coordination they must have with the other field groups. The Field Sampling Group will normally include an Air Monitoring Team, Water Sampling Team, and a Soil Sampling Team. They will normally be responsible for perimeter monitoring and sampling, and will either coordinate sampling within the hot zone and warm zones with the Entry Group, or if properly trained and outfitted with PPE, they may take samples within the hot/warm zones themselves. They will be responsible for:

a. Conducting all sampling required for immediate operation activity and communicating sampling data, such as results of routine air monitoring to on-site operational and safety personnel.

b. Conducting air, water, and soil sampling as directed by the regulatory agencies and other interested parties through the Sampling Protocol Team.

c. Ensuring that all samples are obtained following appropriate sample protocol and other special instructions they may obtain.

d. Ensuring that all samples taken are properly documented and following the chain of custody procedures.

e. Ensuring that the samples are properly transferred to the Sample Documentation and Tracking Teams for proper documentation, analysis, and final dissemination.

SCIENTIFIC SUPPORT COORDINATOR SPECIALIST
- The Scientific Support Coordinator (SSC) is a technical specialist and is defined in the NCP as the principal advisor to the FOSC for scientific issues. The SSC is responsible for providing expertise on chemical hazards, field observations, trajectory analysis, resources at risk, environmental trade-offs of countermeasures and cleanup methods, and information management. The SSC is also charged with gaining consensus on scientific issues affecting the response and ensuring that differing opinions within the scientific community are communicated to the IC/UC. Additionally, the SSC is responsible for providing data on weather, tides, and currents, and other applicable environmental conditions. The SSC can serve as the Environmental Unit Leader.

  a. Review Common Responsibilities in Chapter 2.
  b. Attend planning meetings.
  c. Determine resource needs.
  d. Provide overflight maps and trajectory analysis to the Situation Unit.
  e. Provide weather, tidal and current information.
  f. Obtain consensus on scientific issues affecting the response.
  g. Develop a prioritized list of the resources at risk.
  h. Provide information on chemical hazards.
  i. Evaluate environmental tradeoffs of countermeasures and cleanup methods, and response endpoints.
  j. Maintain Unit Log (ICS 214-CG).

TECHNICAL SPECIALIST GROUP SUPERVISOR -
There are a number of specialist positions that will be required for hazardous substance response operations. Because of their field locations and requirement for close coordination with the Operations Section Field Personnel, they are assigned to the Technical Group.

HAZARDOUS SUBSTANCE   HAZARDOUS SUBSTANCE

The Technical Specialist Group Supervisor is responsible for coordinating the activities of these various specialists and ensuring that their services and information are made available to the appropriate field and command post activities. The Technical Group Supervisor will:

a. Review the Division/Group Supervisor responsibilities in Chapter 7.
b. Will oversee the activities of the following identified specialists.

TECHNICAL SPECIALIST-HAZARDOUS SUBSTANCE/MATERIALS REFERENCE - This

position provides technical information and assistance to the Hazardous Substances/Material Group using various reference sources such as computer databases, technical journals, CHEMTREC, and phone contact with facility representatives. The Technical Specialist Hazardous Substances/Materials Reference may provide product identification using hazardous categorization tests and/or any other means of identifying unknown materials.

a. Review Common Responsibilities in Chapter 2.
b. Obtain a briefing from the PSC.
c. Provide technical support to the Hazardous Substance/Materials Group Supervisor.
d. Maintain communications and coordinate operations with the Entry Leader.
e. Provide and interpret environmental monitoring information.
f. Provide analysis of hazardous material samples. Determine PPE compatibility to hazardous material.
g. Provide technical information of the incident for documentation.
h. Provide technical information management with public and private agencies (i.e.; Poison Control

Center, Toxicology Center, CHEMTREC, State
Department of Food and Agriculture, National
Response Team).

i.   Assist the Planning Section with projecting the
     potential environmental effects of the release.
j.   Maintain Unit Log (ICS 214-CG).

TOXICOLOGIST – The Toxicologist Specialist is a
trained, certified professional that can determine the
toxic effects of the released hazardous substance on
responders, the public, and the environment. This
position is required by regulation for Coast Guard
approved FRP and VRP and will be on-scene on behalf
of the RP.

INDUSTRIAL HYGIENIST – An Industrial Hygienist
Specialist is a trained and certified professional that can
assist the SOFR in determining appropriate protective
measures to be taken by responders in complex
hazardous substances responses to ensure the workers
health and safety.

CHEMICAL ENGINEER – A Chemical Engineer is a
trained and licensed professional that is knowledgeable
in the development and application of manufacturing
processes in which materials undergo changes in
properties and that deals especially with the design and
operation of plants and equipment to perform such
work.

PRODUCT EXPERT – The Product Expert is a trained
professional that is knowledgeable about the specific
hazardous substance product that is released, and in
particular the chemical changes that may occur when it
is released into the environment, such as water, air, etc.

MARINE CHEMIST – A Marine Chemist Specialist is a

trained professional, usually a chemist or industrial hygienist certified for declaring confined spaces as gas free for entry.

ASSISTING AGENCIES

LAW ENFORCEMENT – The local law enforcement agency will respond to most Hazardous Substance/Material incidents. Depending on incident factors, law enforcement may be a partner in UC or may participate as an assisting agency. Some functional responsibilities that may be handled by law enforcement are:

a. Isolate the incident area.
b. Manage crowd control.
c. Manage traffic control.
d. Manage public protective action.
e. Provide scene management for on-highway incidents.
f. Manage criminal investigations.

ENVIRONMENTAL HEALTH AGENCIES – In most cases the local or State environmental health agency will be at the scene as a partner in UC. Some functional responsibilities that may be handled by environmental health agencies are:

a. Determine the identity and nature of the Hazardous Substances/Materials.
b. Establish the criteria for clean up and disposal of the Hazardous Substances/Materials.
c. Declare the site safe for re-entry by the public.
d. Provide the medical history of exposed individuals.
e. Monitor the environment.
f. Supervise the clean up of the site.
g. Enforce various laws and acts.
h. Determine legal responsibility.

20-29

HAZARDOUS SUBSTANCE   **HAZARDOUS SUBSTANCE**

i. Provide technical advice.
j. Approve funding for the clean up, if required.

TECHNICAL SPECIALISTS

SAMPLING PROTOCOL TEAM - During a significant hazardous substance/Material release incident, there will be numerous requirements for sampling under the ICS UC umbrella. Unless control is taken immediately, there is the possibility for each entity with regulatory or legal interest to begin a sampling regimen independent of each other. The Sampling Protocol team under the Planning Section would be responsible for:

a. Determining the overall sampling protocol for the incident.
b. Coordinating within the interested parties what analysis is required for overall samples.
c. Coordinating procedures for split samples between all parties.
d. Providing special instructions to the field sampling teams operating under the OPS.
e. Coordinate with appropriate agencies and the RP, and determine independent laboratories to be used for analysis, and coordinating the contracting of their services with the Logistics Section and Finance Section.
f. Providing specific special instructions to the laboratories for analytical work.

SAMPLE TRACKING TEAM – As indicated above for sample documentation, there is the possibility of thousands of samples to be taken for analysis during a significant hazardous substance release incident. The Sample Tracking Team will be responsible for:

a. Ensuring that all samples are collected from Field Sampling Teams.
b. Coordinate preferred turn around times for

20-30

HAZARDOUS SUBSTANCE   HAZARDOUS SUBSTANCE

specific samples being analyzed.
c. Ensuring that proper chain of custody documents are prepared and logged for all samples.
d. Assign control numbers to all samples.
e. Ensure samples are properly transferred to the appropriate laboratory, and documented.
f. Track samples to ensure that sample analysis are completed according to requested schedule, and determine reasons for delays.

SAMPLE DISSEMINATION TEAM – During a significant Hazardous Substance release there are many occasions when several parties will need the information obtained from a sample analysis. It will be the responsibility of this team to ensure that all parties with a legitimate need for a copy of an analysis obtain it as soon as the information is available. They will coordinate this activity with the Sample Documentation Team and the Sample Tracking Team to ensure that the original analysis document is retained in the Documentation Section for the historical event file.

HUMAN HEALTH ASSESSMENT TEAM – The effects of the release on human health will be a primary concern during the incident. The Human Health Assessment Team will be responsible for:
a. Coordinating activities involving the release to determine the risk to humans, including acute and chronic public health threats, and to advise the UC on their findings.
b. They will coordinate and provide advice to city/county and state health agencies having responsibility for human and public health.

CLEANUP TECHNICAL TEAM – During the emergency phase of the release incident, the primary goal for the operation will be to secure the source of the release, and to minimize effects of the release on the public and environment. These efforts will usually involve firefighting, plugging and patching tanks, evacuation of threatened persons, search and rescue, etc. However, it is important that while these efforts are in progress, work begins on determining appropriate cleanup methods for the effected areas. This team will:

a. Research the state of the art approaches for mitigating the hazardous substance product released.

b. Determine the most reasonable and economical approach for remediating the effects of the release.

c. Determine the most qualified and reasonable contractor(s) for accomplishing the remediation work and coordinate obtaining their services with the Logistics and Finance Sections.

d. Develop a Remediation Plan for approval by the UC.

e. Review information obtained throughout the emergency phase, and modify the remediation plan as required so it is up to date at the time of implementation.

CHAPTER 21

MARINE FIRE

CHAPTER 21

MARINE FIRE

References:
  (a) National Response Plan (NRP)
  (b) National Incident Management System (NIMS)

INTRODUCTION

The marine fire chapter is designed to provide an
organization structure that will provide supervision and
control for the essential functions required at marine fire
incidents. The response and organizational structure to
a marine fire can vary widely depending on the location
of the vessel and proximity to fire fighting resources,
capabilities of the municipal and industrial fire
departments, type of vessel, and nature of the cargo
and source of the fire.

UNIFIED COMMAND
A marine fire can bring together a variety of entities
depending on the variables discussed above. Although
the Coast Guard does not directly conduct fire fighting, it
does have a major role in coordination and support. For
this reason, a vessel fire would most likely be managed
under UC. A marine fire could bring to the scene fire
departments, law enforcement, public health, technical
cargo experts, industrial fire departments, and private
fire fighting and salvage experts. If pollution and
hazardous materials were involved, the agencies and
complexity would escalate dramatically.

MARINE FIRE SCENARIO AND MODULAR ORGANIZATION DEVELOPMENT

MODULAR DEVELOPMENT - A series of examples of modular development are included to illustrate methods of expanding the incident organization.

INITIAL RESPONSE ORGANIZATION - The first to arrive Fire Department Company Officer will assume command of the incident as the IC. The IC will assume all Command and General Staff functions and responsibilities and manages initial response resources. See Page 21-4 for an example of the Initial Response Organization.

TRANSITIONED RESPONSE ORGANIZATION - The Coast Guard and Fire Department IC have met and established a UC. They have established Fire and Medical Groups. Waterborne resources have arrived and a SOFR has been assigned. See Page 21-5 for an example of the Transitioned Response Organization.

MULTI-DIVISION/GROUP ORGANIZATION - The UC has activated most Command and General Staff positions and has established a combination of divisions and groups. A water division and land staging area have been established. See Page 21-6 for an example of the Multi-Division/Group Organization.

MULTI-ALARM ORGANIZATION - The UC has activated all Command and General Staff positions and has established multiple divisions. Branches would be created if span of control issues warranted. Water staging and stability/salvage groups were implemented. A Coast Guard Officer may serve as Deputy OSC. See Page 21-7 for an example of a Multi-Alarm Organization.

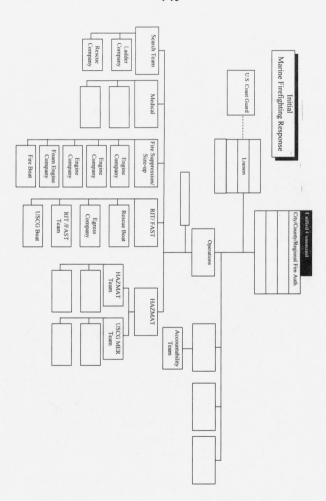

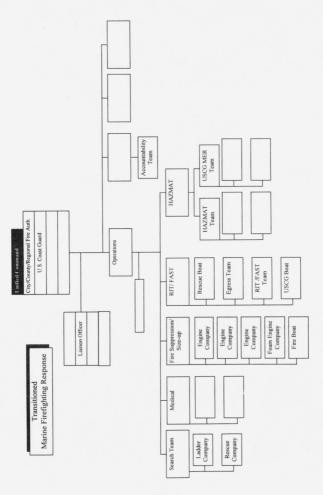

Transitioned Marine Firefighting Response

21-5

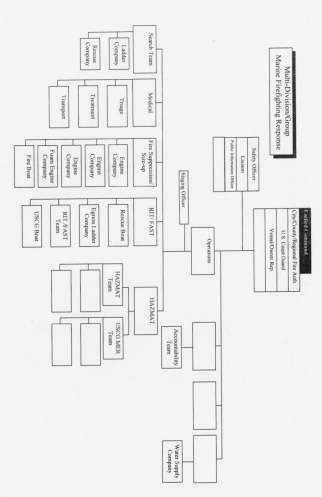

Multi-Division/Group
Marine Firefighting Response

Unified Command
City/County/Regional Fire Auth.
U.S. Coast Guard
Vessel/Owner Rep.

Safety Officer
Liaison
Public Information Officer

Staging Officer

Operations

Accountability Team

Water Supply Company

Fire Suppression/Size-up
Engine Company
Engine Company
Engine Company
Foam Engine Company
Fire Boat

Search Team
Ladder Company
Rescue Company

Medical
Triage
Treatment
Transport

RIT/FAST
Rescue Boat
Egress Ladder Company
RIT/FAST Team
USCG Boat

HAZMAT
HAZMAT Team
USCG MER Team

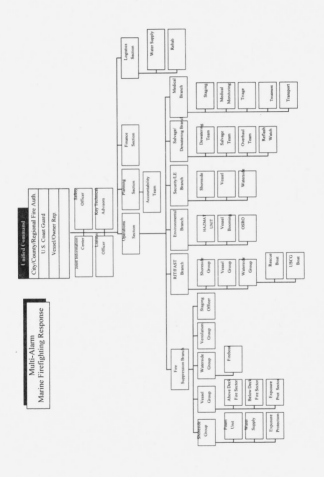

MARINE FIRE SPECIFIC ICS POSITIONS AND TASK DESCRIPTIONS

Only those ICS positions and tasks specific and unique to Marine Firefighting missions will be described in this section. Persons assigned the common positions consistent with the NIMS organization should refer to the position job aids and Chapters 5 through 11 of this Manual for their position/task descriptions and checklists.

ACCOUNTABILITY TEAM – The Accountability Team is responsible for signing in and out all personnel that board a vessel. There must be team members at each entry point to log the entry and exit of all personnel that board the vessel during an incident. Accountability for all resources is the responsibility of the IC/UC and is typically delegated to the Planning Section.

FIRE SUPPRESSION BRANCH - The Fire Suppression Branch Director, when activated, is under the direction of the OSC. The Fire Department's initial Operations Section Chief at a maritime fire is often re-designated the Fire Suppression Branch Director under a UC. The Director is responsible for the assigned portion of the IAP that deals with fire suppression activities, assignment of resources within the branch, and reporting progress of control activities, and status of resources within the branch.

SHORESIDE DIVISION - The Shoreside Division Supervisor is responsible for all shoreside fire suppression activities under the Fire Suppression Branch. The supervisor is responsible for the assigned portion of the IAP that deals with fire suppression activities and exposure protection on shore, assignment of resources within the division, and reporting progress

21-8

of control of activities, and status of resources within the division.

VESSEL DIVISION - The Vessel Division Supervisor is responsible for all vessel fire suppression activities under the Fire Suppression Branch. The supervisor is responsible for the assigned portion of the IAP that deals with fire suppression activities and exposure protection on a vessel, assignment of resources within the division, and reporting progress of control of activities, and status of resources within the division.

WATERSIDE DIVISION - The Waterside Division Supervisor is responsible for all waterside fire suppression activities under the Fire Suppression Branch. The supervisor is responsible for the assigned portion of the IAP that deals with fire suppression activities and exposure protection on the water, assignment of resources within the division, and/or group, and reporting progress of control of activities and status of resources within the division and/or group. This includes all fireboat activities.

VENTILATION GROUP - The Ventilation Group Supervisor is responsible for coordination of vessel CO_2 suppression systems, coordinating the securing of ventilation, use of positive and/or negative pressure ventilation strategies in coordination with the vessel's crew, as required by the Fire Suppression Branch Director reference in the IAP.

RAPID INTERVENTION TEAM - The Rapid Intervention Team (RIT) is contingency team responsible for performing search and rescue of trapped or injured fire fighters. A RIT will normally be assigned in each area the fire activities are taking place, including Shoreside, Vessel and Waterside Branches. On a vessel, a RIT

21-9

will be assigned at each separate entry point where below deck activities are being conducted. The RIT leader is responsible for the assigned portion of the IAP that deals with fire fighter rescue activities.

RIT TEAM LEADER – The RIT Team Leader is responsible for development and implementation of rescue strategies pertaining to each assigned area.

SALVAGE/DEWATERING BRANCH - The Salvage/Dewatering Branch Director, when activated, is under the supervision of the OSC. This branch is responsible for development of a plan to stabilize the vessel, identify equipment/resources needed, and remove water that is being used in suppression activities. The Salvage/Dewatering Branch should be established as soon as firefighting activities are initiated to ensure control of vessel stability. The Salvage/Dewatering Branch Director is responsible for the assigned portion of the IAP that deals with salvage and dewatering activities, the status of assigned resources within the Branch, and reporting progress to the OSC.

DEWATERING TASK FORCE - The Dewatering Task Force is responsible for implementing the dewatering plan developed for the incident. This may include pumping water using portable pumps, draining of water through scuppers made in the vessel, or transferring water to other areas of the vessel.

SITUATIONS REQUIRING SPECIAL ATTENTION

There will be times where special situations develop that will require actions at either a reduced or more elevated level than the previously addressed conditions. In order to facilitate understanding of these situations brief descriptions are provided without organizational structure charts. The descriptions in this section will address several of the situations that have been identified.

MARITIME INCIDENT RESPONSE TEAM – ADVANCE MFF RESPONSE TEAM:

There will be incidents where the Coast Guard will be notified of a fire that may or may not have been contained by the crew on board a vessel enroute to a local port. This will provide the Coast Guard and Fire Department the opportunity to plan for the response. It is often advantageous to send an Advance MFF Response Team to the vessel as soon as possible, and PRIOR to it entering port. This will permit the UC to collect the information needed to make informed decisions, to mitigate the impact of incident, and have adequate appropriate resources available prior to the vessel entering port. The nature of the incident will determine the specific makeup of the team and equipment needed for evaluation.

MULTI-JURSIDICTIONAL RESPONSE – UNIFIED COMMAND:

There may be incidents that, due to the magnitude of the fire or outside influences (e.g. flood, earthquake, hurricane), extend the fire incident outside the original jurisdiction. This will require the rapid establishment of a UC and organization that includes all affected states, counties, jurisdictions, agencies, and organizations. While this organization will be very similar to the Oil Spill response organizations listed in Chapter 19, the rapid spread of fire into other jurisdictions requires an organization that can manage often limited and scarce specialized resources, within a region, and/or in a timely fashion. Establishment of appropriate divisions, groups, and branches will be required to coordinate activities over a large area.

CHAPTER 22

MULTI-CASUALTY

TABLE OF CONTENTS

CHAPTER 22

MULTI-CASUALTY

References:
  (a) National Response Plan (NRP)
  (b) National Incident Management System (NIMS)
  (c) IMO/ICAO International Aeronautical and
      Maritime Search & Rescue Manual, Vols. I & II
  (d) U.S. National Search and Rescue Supplement
      to the International Aeronautical and Maritime
      Search & Rescue Manual
  (e) National Search and Rescue Plan, 1999
  (f) Addendum to the National Search and
      Research Manual, COMDTINST 16130.2
      (series)

INTRODUCTION

The Coast Guard may become involved in various
incidents where the casualty may result in the need to
handle numerous medical patients or victims. This
situation may apply to any of the incidents covered in
the previous chapters. The Multi-Casualty Branch
Structure is designed to provide the Incident
Commander with a basic expandable system for
handling any number of patients in a multi-casualty
incident.

One or more additional Medical Group/Divisions may be
established under the Multi-Casualty Branch Director, if
geographical or incident conditions warrant. The
degree of implementation will depend upon the
complexity of the incident.

MULTI-CASUALTY SCENARIO AND MODULAR ORGANIZATION DEVELOPMENT

MODULAR DEVELOPMENT

A series of examples of modular development are included to illustrate one possible method of expanding the incident organization to deal with multi-casualty, mass patient and victim incidents.

INITIAL RESPONSE ORGANIZATION

Initial response resources are managed by the IC who will handle all Command and General Staff responsibilities. The first arriving resource with the appropriate communications capability should establish communications with the appropriate hospital or other coordinating facility and become the Medical Communications Coordinator. Other first arriving resources would become triage personnel. See Page 22-5 for an example of the Initial Response Organization.

REINFORCED RESPONSE ORGANIZATION

In addition to the initial response, the IC designates a Triage Supervisor, a Treatment Supervisor, Treatment Teams and a Ground Ambulance Coordinator. See Page 22-6 for an example of the Reinforced Response Organization.

MULTI-LEADER RESPONSE ORGANIZATION

The IC has now established an OSC who has in turn established a Medical Supply Coordinator, a Manager for each treatment category and a Patient Transportation Group Supervisor. The Patient Transportation Group Supervisor was needed in order for the OSC to maintain a manageable span of control, based on the assumption that other operations are concurrently happening in the Operations Section. See

Page 22-7 for an example of the Multi-Leader Response Organization.

MULTI-GROUP RESPONSE ORGANIZATION
All positions within the Medical Group and Patient Transportation Group are now filled. The Air Operations Branch is shown to illustrate the coordination between the Air Ambulance Coordinator and the Air Operations Branch. An Extrication Group is freeing trapped victims. See Page 22-8 for an example of the Multi-Group Response Organization.

COMPLETE INCIDENT RESPONSE ORGANIZATION
The complete incident response organization shows the Multi-Casualty Branch and other Branches with which there may be interaction. The Multi-Casualty Branch now has three (3) Medical Divisions (geographically separate), but only one Patient Transportation Group. This is because all patient transportation must be coordinated through one point to avoid overloading hospitals or other medical facilities. See Page 22-9 for an example of the Complete Incident Response Organization.

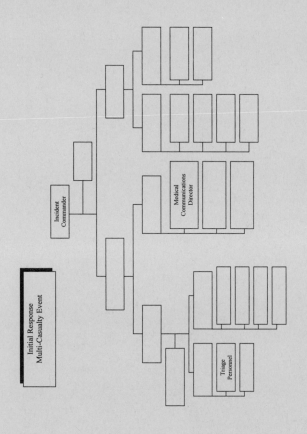

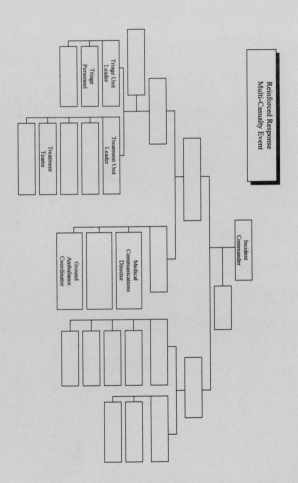

Reinforced Response
Multi-Casualty Event

Incident
Commander

Medical
Communications
Director

Ground
Ambulance
Coordinator

Triage Unit
Leader

Triage
Personnel

Treatment Unit
Leader

Treatment
Teams

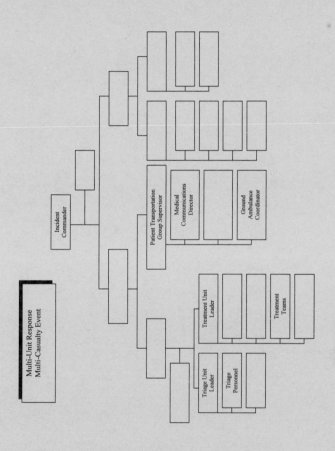

Multi-Unit Response
Multi-Casualty Event

Incident Commander

Patient Transportation Group Supervisor

Medical Communications Director

Ground Ambulance Coordinator

Treatment Unit Leader

Treatment Teams

Triage Unit Leader

Triage Personnel

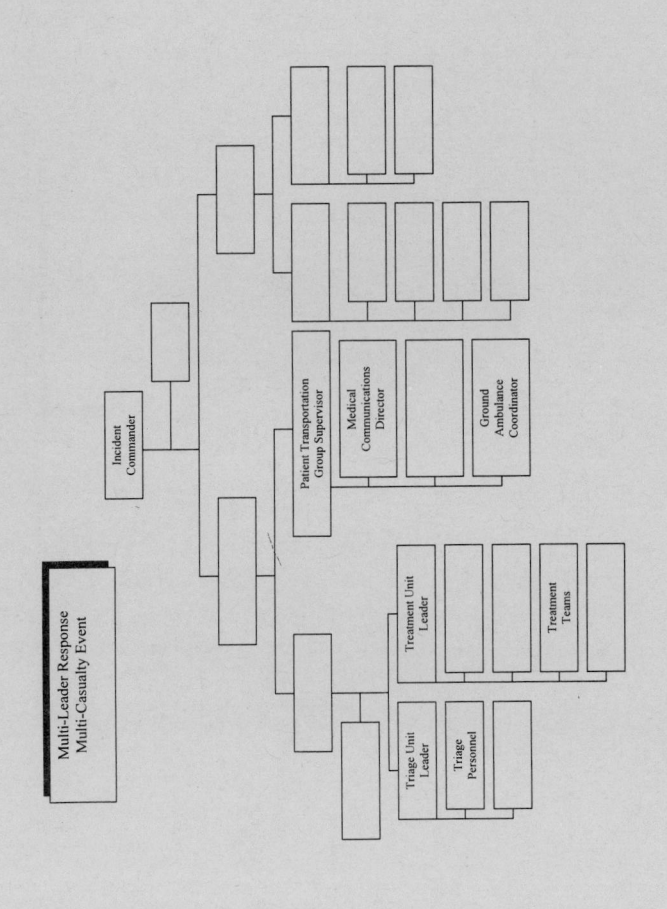

Multi-Leader Response
Multi-Casualty Event

Incident Commander

Patient Transportation Group Supervisor

Medical Communications Director

Ground Ambulance Coordinator

Treatment Unit Leader

Treatment Teams

Triage Unit Leader

Triage Personnel

22-8

MULTI-CASUALTY

MULTI-CASUALTY

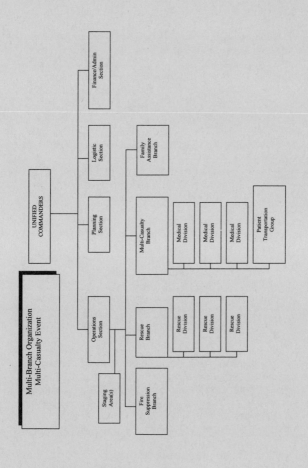

Multi-Branch Organization
Multi-Casualty Event

UNIFIED COMMANDERS

Operations Section

Planning Section

Logistic Section

Finance/Admin Section

Staging Area(s)

Fire Suppression Branch

Rescue Branch

Multi-Casualty Branch

Family Assistance Branch

Rescue Division

Rescue Division

Rescue Division

Medical Division

Medical Division

Medical Division

Patient Transportation Group

MULTI-CASUALTY SPECIFIC ICS POSITIONS AND TASK DESCRIPTIONS

Only those ICS positions and tasks specific and unique to multi-casualty missions will be described in this section. Persons assigned the common positions consistent with the NIMS organization should refer to the position job aids and Chapters 5 through 11 of this Manual for their position/task descriptions and checklists.

MULTI-CASUALTY BRANCH DIRECTOR - The Multi-Casualty Branch Director is responsible for the implementation of the IAP within the Branch. This includes the direction and execution of branch planning for the assignment of resources within the Branch.
   a. Review Branch Director Responsibilities in Chapter 7.
   b. Review Group/Division Assignments for effectiveness of current operations and modify as needed.
   c. Provide input to OSC for the IAP.
   d. Supervise Branch Activities.
   e. Maintain Unit Log (ICS 214-CG).

MEDICAL GROUP/DIVISION SUPERVISOR - The Medical Group/Division Supervisor supervises the Triage Team Leader, Treatment Team Leader and Medical Supply Coordinator. The Medical Group/Division Supervisor establishes command and controls the activities within a Medical Group/Division, in order to assure the best possible emergency medical care to patients during a multi-casualty incident.
   a. Review Division Group responsibilities in Chapter 7.
   b. Participate in Multi-Casualty Branch/Operations Section Planning Activities.

c. Establish Medical Group/Division with assigned personnel. Request additional personnel and resources sufficient to handle the magnitude of the incident.

d. Designate Treatment Team Leaders and treatment area locations as appropriate.

e. Isolate Morgue and Minor Treatment Area from Immediate and Delayed Treatment Areas.

f. Request law enforcement/coroner involvement as needed.

g. Determine amount and types of additional medical resources and supplies needed to handle the magnitude of the incident (medical caches, backboards, litters, cots).

h. Establish communications and coordination with the Patient Transportation Group Supervisor.

i. Ensure activation of hospital alert system, local EMS/health agencies.

j. Direct and/or supervise on-scene personnel from agencies such as Coroner's Office, Red Cross, law enforcement, ambulance companies, county health agencies, and hospital volunteers.

k. Ensure proper security, traffic control, and access for the Medical Group/Division area.

l. Direct medically trained personnel to the appropriate team leader.

m. Maintain Unit Log. (ICS 214-CG).

TRIAGE TEAM LEADER - The Triage Team Leader supervises Triage Personnel/Litter Bearers and the Morgue Manager. The Triage Team Leader assumes responsibility for providing triage management and movement of patients from the triage area. When triage has been completed, the Triage Team Leader may be reassigned as needed.

a. Review Common Responsibilities in Chapter 2.

   b.   Develop organization sufficient to handle assignment.

   c.   Inform Medical Group/Division Supervisor of resource needs.

   d.   Implement triage process.

   e.   Coordinate movement of patients from the Triage Area to the appropriate Treatment Area.

   f.   Give periodic status reports to the Medical Group/Division Supervisor.

   g.   Maintain security and control of the Triage Area.

   h.   Establish Morgue.

TRIAGE PERSONNEL - Triage Personnel appropriately treat patients on-scene and assign them to treatment areas.

   a.   Review Common Responsibilities in Chapter 2.

   b.   Report to designated on-scene triage location.

   c.   Triage and tag injured patients. Classify patients while noting injuries and vital signs if taken.

   d.   Direct movement of patients to proper Treatment Areas.

   e.   Provide appropriate medical treatment (ABC's) to patients prior to movement as incident conditions dictate.

TREATMENT TEAM LEADER - The Treatment Team Leader supervises the Treatment Managers and the Treatment Dispatch Manager. The Treatment Team Leader assumes responsibility for treatment, preparation for transport, and coordination of patient treatment in the Treatment Areas and directs movement of patients to loading location(s).

   a.   Review Common Responsibilities in Chapter 2.

   b.   Develop organization sufficient to handle assignment.

   c.   Direct and supervise Treatment Dispatch, Immediate Delayed, and Minor Treatment Areas.

    d.   Coordinate movement of patients from Triage Area to Treatment Areas with Triage Team Leader.

    e.   Request sufficient medical caches and supplies as necessary.

    f.   Establish communications and coordination with Patient Transportation Group.

    g.   Ensure continual triage of patients throughout Treatment Areas.

    h.   Direct movement of patients to ambulances loading area(s).

    i.   Give periodic status reports to Medical Group/Division Supervisor.

TREATMENT DISPATCH MANAGER - The Treatment Dispatch Manager is responsible for coordinating with Patient Transportation Group, the transportation of patients out of the Treatment Area.

    a.   Review Common Responsibilities in Chapter 2.

    b.   Establish communications with the Immediate, Delayed, and Minor Treatment Managers.

    c.   Establish communications with Patient Transportation Group.

    d.   Verify that patients are prioritized for transportation.

    e.   Advise Medical Communications Coordinator of patient readiness and priority for dispatch.

    f.   Coordinate transportation of patients with the Medical Communications Coordinator.

    g.   Assure that appropriate patient tracking information is recorded.

    h.   Coordinate ambulance loading with Treatment Manager and ambulance personnel.

IMMEDIATE TREATMENT MANAGER - The Immediate Treatment Manager is responsible for

treatment and re-triage of patients assigned to
Immediate Treatment Area.
  a. Review Common Responsibilities in Chapter 2.
  b. Request or establish Medical Teams as
     necessary.
  c. Assign treatment personnel to patients received in
     the Immediate Treatment Area.
  d. Ensure treatment of patients triaged to the
     Immediate Treatment Area.
  e. Assure that patients are prioritized for
     transportation.
  f. Coordinate transportation of patients with
     Treatment Dispatch Manager.
  g. Notify Treatment Dispatch Manager of patient
     readiness and priority for transportation.
  h. Assure that appropriate patient information is
     recorded.

DELAYED TREATMENT MANAGER - The Delayed
Treatment Manager is responsible for treatment and re-
triage of patients assigned to the Delayed Treatment
Area.
  a. Review Common Responsibilities in Chapter 2.
  b. Request or establish Medical Teams as
     necessary.
  c. Assign treatment personnel to patients received in
     the Delayed Treatment Area.
  d. Assure that patients are prioritized for
     transportation.
  e. Coordinate transportation of patients with
     Treatment Dispatch Manager.
  f. Notify Treatment Dispatch Manager of patient
     readiness and priority for transportation.
  g. Assure that appropriate patient information is
     recorded.

MINOR TREATMENT MANAGER - The Minor
Treatment Manager is responsible for treatment and re-triage of patients assigned to the Minor Treatment Area.

   a. Review Common Responsibilities in Chapter 2.

   b. Request or establish Medical Teams as necessary.

   c. Assign treatment personnel to patients received in the Minor Treatment Area.

   d. Assure that patients are prioritized for transportation.

   e. Coordinate transportation of patients with Treatment Dispatch Manager.

   f. Notify Treatment Dispatch Manager of patient readiness and priority for transportation.

   g. Assure that appropriate patient information is recorded.

   h. Coordinate volunteer personnel/organizations through Agency Representatives and Treatment Team Leader.

PATIENT TRANSPORTATION GROUP SUPERVISOR
The Patient Transportation Group Supervisor supervises the Medical Communications Coordinator and the Air and Ground Ambulance Coordinators. The Patient Transportation Group Supervisor is responsible for the coordination of patient transportation and maintenance of records relating to patient identification, injuries, mode of off-incident transportation and destination.

   a. Review Common Responsibilities in Chapter 2.

   b. Review Division Group Supervisor responsibilities in Chapter 7.

   c. Establish communications with hospital(s).

   d. Designate ambulance staging area(s).

   e. Direct the transportation of patients as determined by Treatment Team Leaders.

   f.   Assure that patient information and destination is recorded.
   g. Establish communications with Ambulance Coordinator(s).
   h. Request additional ambulances, as required.
   i.   Notify Ambulance Coordinator(s) of ambulance requests.
   j.   Coordinate requests for air ambulance transportation through the Air Operations Director.
   k. Establish Air Ambulance Helispot with the Multi-Casualty Branch Director and Air Operation Director.
   l.   Maintain Unit Log (ICS 214-CG).

MEDICAL COMMUNICATION COORDINATOR - The Medical Communications Coordinator supervises the Transportation Recorder and maintains communications with the hospital alert system and/or other medical facilities to assure proper patient transportation and destination. The Medical Communication Coordinator coordinates information through the Patient Transportation Group Supervisor and the Transportation Recorder.

   a. Review Common Responsibilities in Chapter 2.
   b. Establish communications with hospital alert system.
   c. Determine and maintain current status of hospital/medical facility availability and capability.
   d. Receive basic patient information and injury status from Treatment Dispatch Manager.
   e. Communicate hospital availability to Treatment Dispatch Manager.
   f.   Coordinate patient off-incident destination with the hospital alert system.
   g. Communicate patient transportation needs to the Ambulance Coordinators based upon requests from Treatment Dispatch Manager.

h. Maintain appropriate records.

AIR/GROUND AMBULANCE COORDINATOR - The Air/Ground Ambulance Coordinators are responsible for managing the Air/Ground Ambulance Staging Areas, and for dispatching ambulances as requested.

a. Review Common Responsibilities in Chapter 2
b. Establish appropriate staging area for ambulances.
c. Establish routes of travel for ambulances for incident operations.
d. Establish and maintain communications with the Air Operations Branch Director.
e. Establish and maintain communications with the Medical Communications Coordinator and the Treatment Dispatch Manager. Provide ambulances upon request from the Medical Communications Coordinator.
f. Maintain records as required.
g. Assure that necessary equipment is available in the ambulance for patient needs during transportation.
h. Establish immediate contact with ambulance agencies at the scene.
i. Request additional transportation resources as appropriate.
j. Provide an inventory of medical supplies at the ambulance staging area for use at the scene.

FAMILY ASSISTANCE BRANCH – The Family Assistance Branch provides services to the victims' family members; coordinates activities, lodging, food, spiritual and emotional needs, and transportation to special events (press conferences, memorial services to the scene of the incident when authorized, etc.), and any special needs that arise during the incident that may assist the victims' family members. NOTE: The

22-17

National Transportation Safety Board (NTSB) typically provides this assistance for major transportation disasters.

The major responsibilities of the Family Assistance Branch are:

a. Review Common Responsibilities in Chapter 2.

b. Review Branch Director responsibilities in Chapter 7.

c. Coordinate with local and state authorities, to include the medical examiner, local law enforcement, emergency management, hospitals, and other emergency support personnel.

d. Conduct daily coordination meetings with the local and Federal government representatives to review daily activities, resolve problem areas, and synchronize future family support operations and activities.

e. Coordinate and provide briefings to families at the site and those who decide not to be at the site.

f. Ensure adequate number of Family Assistance Team members present at all times to allow for rest, exercise and proper rotation.

g. Establish and maintain working relationship with the CERT and CISM teams to cross-reference needs of the victims' families.

h. Attend all staff briefings and planning meetings as required.

i. Request necessary equipment and supplies through LSC.

j. Ensure adequate lodging and/or sleeping arrangements.

k. Ensure that security needs for the victims' family members are addressed.

l. Ensure that all communications are centrally coordinated.

m. Ensure that all transportation scheduling is centrally coordinated.

22-18

n. Maintain Unit Log (ICS 214-CG).
o. The following agencies provide similar assistance during emergencies and may be of assistance:
   - American Red Cross (ARC)
   - Department of Health and Human Services (DHHS)
   - Federal Emergency Management Agency (FEMA)
   - NTSB

MEDICAL SUPPLY COORDINATOR - The Medical Supply Coordinator is responsible for acquiring and maintaining control of appropriate medical equipment and supplies from units assigned to the Medical Group.
a. Review Common Responsibilities in Chapter 2.
b. Acquire, distribute and maintain status of medical equipment and supplies within the Medical Group/Division.
c. Request additional medical supplies (medical caches). If the Logistics Section is established, the Medical Supply Coordinator will coordinate needs with the Supply Unit Leader.
d. Distribute medical supplies to Treatment and Triage Teams.
e. Maintain Unit Log (ICS 214-CG).

MORGUE MANAGER - The Morgue Manager is responsible for Morgue Area activities until relieved of that responsibility by the Office of the Coroner.
a. Review Common Responsibilities in Chapter 2.
b. Assess resource/supply needs and order as needed.
c. Coordinate all Morgue Area activities.
d. Keep area off limits to all but authorized personnel.

e. Coordinate with law enforcement and assist the Coroners Office as necessary.
f. Keep identity of deceased persons confidential.
g. Maintain appropriate records.
h. Maintain Unit Log (ICS 214-CG).

HOSPITAL EMERGENCY RESPONSE TEAM (HERT)

A Hospital Emergency Response Team is recommended to consist of a minimum of three (3) medical personnel, optimum of five (5) medical personnel, which includes a team leader and any combination of physicians, nurses or physicians' assistants. HERT Teams will be requested through the Incident Commander. HERT Teams report to the Treatment Team Leader and assume responsibility for patient assessment and treatment as assigned.

a. Review Common Responsibilities in Chapter 2.
b. Report to the Incident Command Post for assignment.
c. Perform medical treatment and other duties as assigned.
d. Remain at assigned Treatment Area unless otherwise reassigned.
e. Respond to scene with appropriate emergency medical equipment.
f. Maintain Unit Log (ICS 214-CG).

CHAPTER 23

EVENT MANAGEMENT
AND
NATIONAL SPECIAL SECURITY EVENTS (NSSEs)

TABLE OF CONTENTS

EVENT MANAGEMENT
AND
NATIONAL SPECIAL SECURITY EVENTS (NSSEs)

References:
   (a) Presidential Decision Directive 62 (PDD-62), May
        1998
   (b) Homeland Security Presidential Directive 5
        (HSPD – 5)
   (c) Homeland Security Presidential Directive 7
        (HSPD – 7)
   (d) National Response Plan (NRP)
   (e) National Incident Management System (NIMS)
   (f) Event Management Job Aid

NOTE: This chapter provides a very brief overview of
Natiional Special Security Event (NSSE) and Event
Management. For more information, please see
references (a) through (c).

INTRODUCTION

Event Management is becoming more significant in daily
operations. Planned Events can vary from a local
Opsail to large scale National Special Security Events
(NSSE's) as described in reference (a). Events while in
they may require a significant organization to run; the
possible contingencies associated with events must
also be planned for (such as protests and terrorist
actions). Because of the flexibility and structure of
NIMS ICS, planning and executing Events using NIMS
ICS can make the event run smoother and make
contingency execution simpler.

Presidential Decision Directive 62 (PDD – 62)
established NSSE's as a designated event that by virtue
of its political, economic, social, or religious significance

23-2

may be the target of terrorism or criminal activity. Homeland Security Presidential Directive 5 (HSPD – 5) directs DHS responsibility for domestic incident management and coordination of the Federal Government's operational response resources in preparing for and responding to terrorist attacks. Under Homeland Security Presidential Directive 7 (HSPD-7), the Secretary of DHS will make the final determination to designate an event as an NSSE in consultation with the Homeland Security Council.

The NSSE designation process is initiated by a formal request from the governor of the state hosting the event to the Secretary of the Department of Homeland Security (DHS). In situations where the event is federally sponsored (e.g., State of the Union Address), an appropriate federal official will make the request. Additionally, Secretary DHS retains full authority to directly designate NSSE events.

Formal requests are reviewed by the NSSE Working Group, comprised of representatives from the US Secret Service (USSS), Federal Bureau of Investigation (FBI), DHS Emergency Preparedness and Response (EP&R), Federal Emergency Management Agency (FEMA), Department of Defense (DOD) and other DHS agencies with USCG members from COMDT (G-RPC). The NSSE Working Group provides a consensus recommendation to the Secretary DHS regarding NSSE designation. Factors typically considered:
- Federal participation.
- Anticipated attendance by dignitaries.
- Size, significance, and duration of the event.
- Location and recurring nature of the event.
- Anticipated media coverage.

- State and local resources available to support the event.
- Multiplicity of jurisdictions.
- Adequacy of security absent NSSE designation.
- Available threat assessments.

Once NSSE designation has been made, the USSS contacts the relevant federal, state, and local officials to begin planning, coordinating, and implementing a comprehensive security plan for the event. Events that fail to meet required criteria for NSSE designation are considered Special Event Homeland Security (SEHS) under categorized levels I thru IV. The SEHS Working Group is comprised of all DHS agencies including USCG members from COMDT (G-RPC). The SEHS process is similar to NSSE designation for determining the level and thereby the appropriate support given to an event.

NSSE and SEHS working groups provide lists of designated events to their membership identified on the Prioritized Special Event List compiled by DHS. When COMDT (G-RPC) receives the list of events, the list is then forwarded to the Areas for review and action to continue support as required. A designated Federal Coordinator (FC) directs jointly conducted detailed planning and coordination of all assets and resources allocated from participating organizations throughout event execution until conclusion, by way of submitting a consolidated final report to DHS.

When activated to support an NSSE or other security coordination function, the DHS/U.S. Secret Service (USSS) Multi-agency Command Center (MACC) and the FBI JOC are collocated at the JFO when possible.

These agencies work together using the principles of Unified Command, with a pre-designated PFO facilitating interagency incident management coordination during NSSE planning and execution. For these situations, the JFO combines the functions of the DHS/USSS MACC, the FBI JOC, and the Response and Recovery Operations Branch.

EVENT MANAGEMENT AND
NATIONAL SPECIAL SECURITY EVENT (NSSE)
SPECIFIC ICS POSITIONS AND TASK
DESCRIPTIONS

Figure 9 of the NRP (reference (a)) shows the structure for an NSSE.

For NSSE's, a third branch, the Security Operations Branch, may be added to coordinate protection and security efforts.

Security Operations Branch: The Security Operations Branch coordinates protection and site security efforts, and incorporates the functions of the DHS/USSS MACC during NSSE's.

Multi-agency Command Center (MACC). An interagency coordination center established by DHS/USSS during NSSE's as a component of the JFO. The MACC serves as the focal point for interagency security planning and coordination, including the coordination of all NSSE-related information from other intra-agency centers (e.g., police command posts, Secret Service security rooms) and other interagency centers (e.g., intelligence operations centers, joint information centers).

Operational supplements typically are detailed plans relating to specific incidents or events. Operational supplements routinely are developed to support NSSE's.

NOTE: For more information on Event Management, please see references (a) through (c).

CHAPTER 24

COAST GUARD NIMS ICS FORMS LIST
For Incident Management Team and Area Command
Note: Forms noted with * have NIIMS equivalent forms

Incident Management Team Forms

ICS Form #	Form Title	Prepared By
ICS 201-CG*	Incident Briefing	Initial Incident Commander
ICS 202-CG*	Incident Objectives	Planning Section Chief
ICS 203-CG*	Organization Assignment List	Resources Unit Leader
ICS 204-CG*	Assignment List	Resources Unit Leader & Operations Section Chief
ICS 204a-CG	Assignment List Attachments	Operations & Planning Sections Staff
ICS 205-CG*	Incident Radio Communications Plan	Communications Unit Leader
ICS 205a-CG	Communications List	Communications Unit Leader
ICS 206-CG*	Medical Plan	Medical Unit Leader
ICS 207-CG*	Incident Organization Chart	Resources Unit Leader
ICS-208-CG	Site Safety Plan	Safety Officer
ICS 209-CG	Incident Status Summary	Situation Unit Leader
ICS-210	Status Change Card	On-scene Incident Dispatcher

24-1

ICS Form #	Form Title	Prepared By
ICS 211-CG*	Check-In List	Resources Unit/ Check-in Recorder
ICS 213	General Message	Any message originator
ICS-213 RR CG	Resource Request Message	Any Resource Requester
ICS 214-CG*	Unit Log	All Sections and Units
ICS 215-CG*	Operational Planning Worksheet	Operations Section Chief
ICS 215a-CG	Hazard/Risk Analysis Worksheet	Safety Officer
ICS 218	Support Vehicle/Vessel Inventory	Ground/Vessel Support Unit Leaders
ICS-219	Resource Status Card	Resources Unit Leader
ICS 220-CG*	Air Operations Summary Worksheet	Operations Section Chief or Air Branch Director
ICS 221-CG*	Demobilization Checkout	Demobilization Unit Leader
ICS 230-CG	Daily Meeting Schedule	Situation Unit Leader
ICS 232-CG	Resources at Risk Summary	Environmental Unit Leader
ICS 233-CG	Open Action Tracking	Situation Unit Leader
ICS 234-CG	Work Analysis Matrix	Operations & Planning Section Chiefs

Area Command Team Forms

ICS Form #	Form Title	Prepared By
ICS AC202-CG	Area Command Objectives/Priorities	Planning Section Chief
ICS AC205-CG	Area Command Communications List	Communications Unit Leader
ICS AC207-CG	Area Command Organization Chart	Resource Unit Leader
ICS AC209-CG	Area Command Status Summary	Situation Unit Leader
ICS 211-CG*	Check-in List	Resource Unit Leader
ICS 214-CG*	Unit Log	All Sections and Units
ICS AC215-CG	Resource Allocation & Prioritization Worksheet	Command & Planning Section Chief
ICS AC230-CG	Area Command Daily Meeting Schedule	Situation Unit Leader
ICS 233-CG	Open Action Tracking	Situation Unit Leader
ICS AC235-CG	Area Command Log Of significant Events	Planning Section Chief

THIS PAGE INTENTIONALLY LEFT BLANK

CHAPTER 25

GLOSSARY AND ACRONYMS

ACCESS CONTROL POINT – The point of entry and exit from control zones at a Hazardous Substance Incident. This physical location is controlled by response personnel limiting access to and from work areas.

AGENCY – A division of government with a specific function, or a non-governmental organization.

AGENCY REPRESENTATIVE (AREP) – Individual assigned to an incident from an assisting or cooperating agency that has been delegated full authority to make decisions on all matters affecting their agency's participation at the incident. Agency Representatives report to the incident LNO.

ALL RISK – Any incident or event, natural or human caused, that warrants action to protect life, property, environment, public health or safety to minimize disruption of government, social, or economic activities.

ALL-HAZARD – Any incident or event, natural or human caused, that requires an organized response by a public, private, and/or governmental entity in order to protect life, public health and safety, values to be protected, and to minimize any disruption of governmental, social, and economic services.

ALTERNATIVE RESPONSE TECHNOLOGIES (ART) – Response methods or techniques other than mechanical containment or recovery. ART may include use of chemical dispersants, in-situ burning, bioremediation, or other alternatives. Application of ART must be authorized and directed by the OSC.

AREA COMMAND – An organization established to: (1) oversee the management of multiple incidents that are each being handled by an ICS Incident Management Teams (IMT) organization or (2) oversee the management of large or multiple incidents to which several IMTs have been assigned. Area Command has the responsibility to set overall strategy and priorities, allocate critical resources according to priorities, ensure that incidents are properly managed, and ensure that objectives are met and strategies followed. (See also: Unified Area Command).

ASSIGNED RESOURCES – Resources checked-in and assigned work tasks on an incident.

ASSIGNMENTS – Tasks given to resources to perform within a given operational period, based upon tactical objectives in the IAP.

ASSISTANT – Title for subordinates of the Command Staff positions assigned to assist the Command Staff person manage their workload. In some cases, assistants are also assigned to unit leader positions in the planning, logistics, and finance/administration sections.

ASSISTING AGENCY – Is an agency directly contributing or providing tactical or service resources to another agency.

AVAILABLE RESOURCES – Incident-based resources that are immediately available for assignment.

BASE – That location at which the primary logistics functions are coordinated and administered. (Incident name or other designator will be added to the term "Base.") The ICP may be collocated with the Base. There is only one Base per incident.

BRANCH – The organizational level having functional and/or geographic responsibility for major incident operations. The Branch level is organizationally between Section and Division/Group in the Operations Section and between Section and Units in the Logistics Section. Branches are identified by roman numerals or by functional name (e.g. service, support).

BUYING TEAM – A team that supports incident procurement and is authorized to procure a wide range of services, supplies, and equipment rentals.

CACHE – A pre-determined complement of tools, equipment, and/or supplies stored in a designated location, and available for incident use.

CAMP – Geographical site(s) within the general incident area, separate from the incident base, equipped and staffed to provide sleeping, food, water, and sanitary services to incident personnel.

CHECK-IN – Process whereby resources first report to incident response. Check-in locations include: Incident Command Post (Resources Unit), Incident Base, Camps, Staging Areas, Helibases, Helispots, or Division/Group Supervisors (for direct tactical assignments).

CHIEF – The ICS title for individuals responsible for the command of functional Sections: Operations, Planning, Logistics, and Finance/Administration.

CLEAR TEXT – The use of plain English in radio communications transmission. Neither 10 Codes nor agency-specific codes are used when using Clear Text.

COMMAND – The act of directing, ordering, and/or controlling resources by virtue of explicit legal, agency, or delegated authority. May also refer to an IC or to the UC.

COMMAND POST – See Incident Command Post.

COMMAND STAFF – The Command Staff consists of the PIO, SOFR, and LNO, who report directly to an IC. May also include Intelligence Officer. They may have an assistant or assistants, as needed.

COMMON OPERATING PICTURE – Is a broad view of the overall situation as reflected by situation reports, aerial photography and other information and intelligence.

COMPLEX – Two or more individual incidents located in the same general proximity, which are assigned to a single IC or UC to facilitate management.

CONTAMINANT – See Pollutant.

CONTAMINATION CONTROL LINE (CCL) – The established line around the Contamination Reduction Zone that separates the Contamination Reduction Zone from the Support Zone.

CONTAMINATION REDUCTION CORRIDOR (CRC) – A CRC is that area within the Contamination Reduction Zone where the actual decontamination is to take place. Exit from the Exclusion Zone is through the

Contamination Reduction Corridor (CRC). The CRC will become contaminated as people and equipment pass through to the decontamination stations.

CONTAMINATION REDUCTION ZONE (CRZ) – That area between the Exclusion Zone and the Support Zone. This zone contains the Personnel Decontamination Station. This zone may require a lesser degree of personnel protection than the Exclusion Zone. This area separates the contaminated area from the clean area and acts as a buffer to reduce contamination of the clean area.

CONTINGENCY PLAN – The portion of an IAP or other plan that identifies possible but unlikely events and the contingency resources needed to mitigate those events.

CONTROL ZONES – The geographical areas within the control lines set up at a hazardous substance incident. The three zones most commonly used are the Exclusion Zone, Contamination Reduction Zone, and Support Zone.

COOPERATING AGENCY – An agency supplying assistance other than direct tactical or support functions or resources to the incident control effort (e.g., Red Cross, law enforcement agency, telephone company, etc.).

COORDINATION CENTER – Term used to describe any facility that is used for the coordination of agency or jurisdictional resources in support of one or more incidents.

COST SHARING AGREEMENTS – Agreements between agencies or jurisdictions to share designated costs related to incidents. Cost sharing agreements are normally written but may also be verbal between an authorized agency or jurisdictional representatives at the incident.

CRITICAL INFRASTRUCTURES – Systems and assets, whether physical or virtual, so vital to the United States that the incapacity or destruction of such systems and assets would have a debilitating impact on security, national economic security, national public health or safety, or any combination of those matters.

DEMOBILIZATION – Release of resources from an incident in strict accordance with a detailed plan approved by the IC/UC.

DEPUTY – A fully qualified individual who, in the absence of a superior, could be delegated the authority to manage a functional operation or perform a specific task. In some cases, a Deputy could act as relief for a superior and, therefore, **must be fully qualified** in the position. Deputies can be assigned to the Incident Commander, General Staff, and Branch Directors.

DIRECTOR – ICS title for individuals responsible for supervision of a Branch.

DIVISION – Organization level used to divide an incident into geographical areas of operation. The Division level is established when the number of resources exceeds the span-of-control of the OSC and is organizationally between the Task Force/Team and the Branch. (See also: Group.)

EMERGENCY OPERATIONS CENTER (EOC) – The pre-designated facility established by an agency or jurisdiction to coordinate the overall agency or jurisdictional response and support to an emergency.

The EOC coordinates information and resources to support domestic incident management activities.

EMERGENCY SUPPORT FUNCTION (ESF) – The National Response Plan (NRP) details 15 ESFs in place to coordinate operations during Federal involvement in an incident including transportation, communications, public works, engineering, firefighting, information and planning, mass care, resource support, health and medical services, urban search and rescue, hazardous materials, food, and energy.

EVENT – A planned, non-emergency activity. ICS can be used as the management system for a wide range of events, e.g. NSSES, Opsail, parades, concerts, or sporting activities. The event IAP usually includes contingency plans for possible incidents that might occur during the event.

EXCLUSION ZONE – The area immediately around a spill or release where contamination does or could occur. The innermost of the three zones of a hazardous substance/material incident. Special protection is required for all personnel while in this zone.

EXPANDED ORDERING – An organization that is authorized to set up outside of the ICP to assist the Logistics Section with ordering supplies, services and resources to support the incident. The expanded ordering does not decide allocation of critical resources because they are dealt with by Area Command.

FACILITY OWNER (FO) – FO is the owner/operator of the facility or source which precipitated an incident.

FEDERAL COORDINATING OFFICER (FCO) – The Federal officer who is appointed to manage Federal

25-7

resource support activities related to Stafford Act disasters and emergencies. The FCO is responsible for coordinating the timely delivery of Federal disaster assistance resources and programs to the affected State and local governments, individual victims, and the private sector.

FEDERAL ON-SCENE COORDINATOR (FOSC) – The Federal official pre-designated by the EPA or the USCG to coordinate responses under subpart D of the NCP (40 CFR 300) or the government official designated to coordinate and direct removal actions under subpart E of the NCP. A FOSC can also be designated as the Incident Commander.

FEDERAL RESOURCE COORDINATOR (FRC) – The Federal official appointed to manage Federal resource support activities related to non-Stafford Act incidents. The FRC is responsible for coordinating support from other Federal departments and agencies using interagency agreements and MOU's.

FEDERAL INCIDENT RESPONSE SUPPORT TEAM (FIRST) – A forward component of the ERT-A that provides on-scene support to the local Incident Command or Area Command structure.

FINANCE/ADMINISTRATION SECTION – The section responsible for all administrative and financial considerations on an incident.

GENERAL STAFF – The group of incident management personnel reporting to the IC and are comprised of: OSC, PSC, LSC, and FSC. They may each have a deputy/deputies.

GEOGRAPHIC INFORMATION SYSTEM (GIS) – A GIS is an electronic information system, which provides a geo-referenced database to support management decision-making.

GROUP – An organizational level established to divide the incident into functional areas of operation. Groups are composed of resources assembled to perform a special function not necessarily within a single geographic division. A Group is located between Branches (when activated) and Resources in the Operations Section. (See also: Division)

HAND CREW – A number of individuals that have been organized and trained and are supervised principally for operational assignments on an incident.

HAZARDOUS CATEGORIZATION TEST (HAZ CAT) – A field analysis to determine the hazardous characteristics of an unknown substance.

HAZARDOUS MATERIAL – For the purposes of ESF #1, hazardous material is a substance or material, including a hazardous substance, that has been determined by the Secretary of Transportation to be capable of posing an unreasonable risk to health, safety, and property when transported in commerce, and which has been so designated (see 49 CFR 171.8). For the purposes of ESF #10 and the Oil and Hazardous Materials Incident Annex, the term is intended to mean hazardous substances, pollutants, and contaminants as defined by the NCP.

HAZARDOUS SUBSTANCE – As defined by the NCP, any substance designated pursuant to section 311(b)(2)(A) of the Clean Water Act; any element, compound, mixture, solution, or substance designated pursuant to section 102 of the Comprehensive Environmental Response, Compensation, and Liability Act (CERCLA); any hazardous waste having the characteristics identified under or listed pursuant to section 3001 of the Solid Waste Disposal Act (but not including any waste the regulation of which under the Solid Waste Disposal Act (42 U.S.C. § 6901 et seq.) has been suspended by act of Congress); any toxic pollutant listed under section 307(a) of the Clean Water Act; any hazardous air pollutant listed under section 112 of the Clean Air Act (42 U.S.C. § 7521 et seq.); and any imminently hazardous chemical substance or mixture with respect to which the EPA Administrator has taken action pursuant to section 7 of the Toxic Substances Control Act (15 U.S.C. § 2601 et seq.).

HELIBASE – A location within the general incident area for parking, fueling, maintenance, and loading of helicopters.

HELISPOT – A location where a helicopter can take off and land. Some helispots may be used for temporary loading.

INCIDENT– An occurrence either human-caused or natural phenomenon, that requires action or support by emergency service personnel to prevent or minimize loss of life or damage to property and/or natural resources.

INCIDENT ACTION PLAN (IAP) – An oral or written plan containing general objectives reflecting the overall strategy for managing an incident. It may include the identification of operational resources and assignments. It may also include attachments that provide direction and important information for management of the incident during one or more operational periods.

INCIDENT BASE – Location at the incident where the primary logistics functions are coordinated and administered. The ICP may be collocated with the base. There is only one base per incident.

INCIDENT COMMANDER (IC) – The individual responsible for all incident activities, including the development of strategies and tactics and the ordering and release of resources. The IC has overall authority and responsibility for conducting incident operations and is responsible for the management of all incident operations at the incident site. (See also: Unified Command).

INCIDENT COMMAND POST (ICP) – The field location at which the primary tactical-level, on-scene incident command functions are performed. The ICP may be collocated with the incident base or other incident facilities.

INCIDENT COMMAND SYSTEM (ICS) – A standardized on-scene emergency management concept specifically designed to allow its user(s) to adopt an integrated organizational structure equal to the complexity and demands of single or multiple incidents, without being hindered by jurisdictional boundaries.

INCIDENT MANAGEMENT TEAM (IMT) – The Incident Commander and appropriate Command and General Staff personnel assigned to an incident.

INCIDENT OF NATIONAL SIGNIFICANCE (INS) – An actual or potential high-impact event that requires a coordinated and effective response by an appropriate combination of Federal, State, local, tribal, non-governmental, and/or private-sector entities in order to save lives and minimize damage and provide the basis for long-term community recovery and mitigation activities.

INCIDENT OBJECTIVES – Statements of guidance and direction necessary for the selection of appropriate strategies, and the tactical direction of resources. Tactical incident objectives address the tactical response issues while management incident objectives address the incident management issues. Tactical incident objectives are based on realistic expectations of what can be accomplished when all allocated resources have been effectively deployed. Incident objectives must be achievable and measurable, yet flexible enough to allow for strategic and tactical alternatives.

INCIDENT OVERHEAD – All supervisory positions described in the Incident Command System.

INCIDENT SUPPORT ORGANIZATION – Includes any off-incident support provided to an incident. Examples would be EOCs, airports, expanded ordering, etc.

INCIDENT SITUATION DISPLAY – The Situation Unit is responsible for maintaining a display of status boards, which communicate critical incident information vital to establishing an effective command and control environment.

INITIAL ACTION – The actions taken by the first resources to arrive at the incident. Initial actions may be to size up, patrol, monitor, withhold from any action, or take aggressive initial measures.

INITIAL RESPONSE – Resources initially committed to an incident.

INLAND ZONE – As defined in the NCP, the environment inland of the coastal zone excluding the Great Lakes and specified ports and harbors on the inland rivers. The term "coastal zone" delineates an area of Federal responsibility for response action. Precise boundaries are determined by EPA/USCG agreements and identified in Regional Contingency Plan's (RCPs).

INTELLIGENCE AND INFORMATION – National security, classified information, or other operational information necessary for incident decision making. Traditionally located in the Planning Section but may be moved to other parts of the ICS organization based on Command needs.

JOINT FIELD OFFICE (JFO) – A temporary Federal facility established locally to provide a central point for Federal, State, local, and tribal executives with responsibility for incident oversight, direction, and/or assistance to effectively coordinate protection, prevention, preparedness, response, and recovery actions. The JFO will combine the traditional functions of the JOC, the FEMA DFO, and the JIC within a single Federal facility.

JOINT INFORMATION CENTER (JIC) – A facility established within or near the ICP where the PIO and staff can coordinate and provide information on the incident to the public, media, and other agencies. The JIC is normally staffed with representation from the FOSC, SOSC, and FO.

JOINT INFORMATION SYSTEM (JIS) – Integrates incident information and public affairs into a cohesive organization designed to provide consistent, coordinated, timely information during a crisis or incident operations.

JOINT OPERATIONS CENTER (JOC) – The JOC is the focal point for all Federal investigative law enforcement activities during a terrorist or potential terrorist incident or any other significant criminal incident, and is managed by the SFLEO. The JOC becomes a component of the JFO when the NRP is activated.

JURISDICTION – The range or sphere of authority. Public agencies have jurisdiction at an incident related to their legal responsibilities and authority for incident mitigation. Jurisdictional authority at an incident can be political/geographical (e.g., city, county, state or federal boundary lines) or functional (e.g., police department, health department, etc.). (See also: Multi-jurisdiction Incident.)

LEADER – The ICS title for an individual responsible for a Task Force/Strike Team or functional unit.

LOGISTICS SECTION – The Logistics Section is responsible for providing facilities, services, and materials in support of the incident.

MAJOR DISASTER – As defined by the Stafford Act, any natural catastrophe (including any hurricane, tornado, storm, high water, wind-driven water, tidal wave, tsunami, earthquake, volcanic eruption, landslide, mudslide, snowstorm, or drought) or, regardless of cause, any fire, flood, or explosion, in any part of the United States, which in the determination of the President causes damage of sufficient severity and magnitude to warrant major disaster assistance under this act to supplement the efforts and available resources of States, local governments, and disaster relief organizations in alleviating the damage, loss, hardship, or suffering caused thereby.

MANAGEMENT BY OBJECTIVES – In ICS, this is a top-down management activity which involves the following steps to achieve the incident goal: (1) establishing incident objectives, (2) selection of appropriate strategy(s) to achieve the objectives, and (3) the tactical direction associated with the selected strategy.

MANAGERS – Individuals within ICS organizational units that are assigned specific managerial responsibilities (e.g., Staging Area Manager).

MESSAGE CENTER – The Message Center is part of the Communications Center and collocated with or adjacent to it. It receives, records, and routes information about resources reporting to the incident, resource status, and handles administration, and tactical traffic.

MISSION ASSIGNMENT – The vehicle used by DHS/EPR/FEMA to support Federal operations in a Stafford Act major disaster or emergency declaration. It orders immediate, short-term emergency response assistance when an applicable State or local government is overwhelmed by the event and lacks the capability to perform, or contract for, the necessary work.

MITIGATE – Any action to contain, reduce, or eliminate the harmful effects of a spill or release of a hazardous substance/material.

MOBILIZATION CENTER – An off-incident location at which emergency service personnel and equipment are temporarily located pending assignment, release, or reassignment.

MORGUE (Temporary On-Incident) – Is an area designated for temporary placement of the dead. The Morgue is the responsibility of the Coroner's Office when a Coroner's Representative is on-scene.

MULTI-AGENCY COORDINATION (MAC) – A generalized term which describes the functions and activities of representatives of involved agencies and/or jurisdictions who come together to make decisions regarding the prioritizing of incidents, and the sharing and use of critical resources. The MAC organization is not a part of the on-scene ICS and is not involved in developing incident strategy or tactics.

MULTI-AGENCY INCIDENT – Is an incident where one or more agencies assist a jurisdictional agency or agencies. May be single or Unified Command.

MULTIJURISDICTIONAL INCIDENT – Is an incident requiring action from multiple agencies that each have jurisdiction to manage certain aspects of an incident. In ICS, these incidents will be managed under Unified Command.

NATIONAL INFRASTRUCTURE COORDINATING CENTER (NICC) – Managed by the DHS Information Analysis and Infrastructure Protection Directorate, the NICC monitors the Nation's critical infrastructure and key resources on an ongoing basis. In the event of an incident, the NICC provides a coordinating vehicle to share information with critical infrastructure and key resources information-sharing entities.

NATIONAL RESPONSE CENTER (NRC) – A national communications center for activities related to oil and hazardous substance response actions. The NRC, located at DHS/USCG Headquarters in Washington, DC, receives and relays notices of oil and hazardous substances releases to the appropriate Federal OSC.

NATIONAL RESPONSE PLAN (NRP) – A document that describes the structure and processes comprising a national approach to domestic incident management designed to integrate the efforts and resources of Federal, State, local, tribal, private-sector, and nongovernmental organizations.

NATIONAL RESPONSE SYSTEM (NRS) – Pursuant to the NCP, the NRS is a mechanism for coordinating response actions by all levels of government (40 CFR § 300.21) for oil and hazardous substances spills and releases.

NATIONAL RESPONSE TEAM (NRT) – The NRT, comprised of the 16 Federal agencies with major environmental and public health responsibilities, is the primary vehicle for coordinating Federal agency activities under the NCP. The NRT carries out national planning and response coordination and is the head of a highly organized Federal oil and hazardous substance emergency response network. EPA serves as the NRT Chair, and DHS/USCG serves as Vice Chair.

NATIONAL SPECIAL SECURITY EVENT (NSSE) – A designated event that, by virtue of its political, economic, social, or religious significance, may be the target of terrorism or other criminal activity.

NATIONAL STRIKE FORCE (NSF) – The NSF consists of three strike teams established by DHS/USCG on the Pacific, Atlantic, and Gulf coasts. The strike teams can provide advice and technical assistance for oil and hazardous substances removal, communications support, special equipment, and services.

NOAA WEATHER STATION – A mobile weather data collection and forecasting facility (including personnel) provided by the National Oceanic and Atmospheric Administration (NOAA), which can be utilized within the incident area.

NONGOVERNMENTAL ORGANIZATION (NGO) – A nonprofit entity that is based on interests of its members, individuals, or institutions and that is not created by a government, but may work cooperatively with government to serve a public purpose, i.e., faith-based charity organizations, American Red Cross.

NUCLEAR INCIDENT RESPONSE TEAM (NIRT) – Created by the Homeland Security Act to provide DHS with a nuclear/radiological response capability. When activated, the NIRT consists of specialized Federal response teams drawn from DOE and/or EPA.

OFFICER – The ICS title for personnel responsible for the Command Staff positions of Safety, Liaison, and Public Information.

OPERATIONAL PERIOD – The period of time scheduled for execution of a given set of operation actions as specified in the IAP. Operational Periods can be various lengths, usually not over 24 hours. The Operational Period coincides with the completion of one planning "P" cycle (see Chapter 3 planning cycle).

OPERATIONS COORDINATION CENTER (OCC) – The primary facility of the Multi-Agency Coordination System. It houses staff and equipment necessary to perform MAC functions.

OPERATIONS SECTION – The Section responsible for all operations directly applicable to the primary mission. Directs the preparation of Branch, Division, and/or Unit operational plans, requests or releases resources, makes expedient changes to the IAP as necessary and reports such to the IC.

OUT-OF-SERVICE RESOURCES – Resources assigned to an incident, but they are unable to respond for mechanical, rest, or personnel reasons.

OVERHEAD PERSONNEL – Personnel who are assigned to supervisory positions that includes: Incident Commander, Command Staff, General Staff, Directors, Supervisors, and Unit Leaders.

PERSONAL PROTECTIVE EQUIPMENT (PPE) – That equipment and clothing required to shield or isolate personnel from the chemical, physical, and biological hazards that may be encountered at a hazardous substance/material incident. 33 CFR 154.1026, 33 CFR 155.1026

PLANNING SECTION – The section that is responsible for the collection, evaluation, and dissemination of tactical information related to the incident, and for the preparation and documentation of incident action plans. The section also maintains information on the current and forecasted situation, and on the status of resources assigned to the incident.

POLLUTANT OR CONTAMINANT – As defined in the NCP, includes, but is not limited to, any element, substance, compound, or mixture, including disease-causing agents, which after release into the environment and upon exposure, ingestion, inhalation, or assimilation into any organism, either directly from the environment or indirectly by ingestion through food chains, will or may reasonably be anticipated to cause death, disease, behavioral abnormalities, cancer, genetic mutation, physiological malfunctions, or physical deformations in such organisms or their offspring.

PRINCIPAL FEDERAL OFFICIAL (PFO) – The Federal official designated by the Secretary of Homeland Security to act as his/her representative locally to oversee, coordinate, and execute the Secretary's incident management responsibilities under HSPD-5 for Incidents of National Significance.

QUALIFIED INDIVIDUAL (QI) – The person authorized by the responsible party to act on their behalf, authorize expenditures, and obligate resources.

RADIOLOGICAL EMERGENCY RESPONSE TEAMS (RERT's) – Teams provided by EPA's Office of Radiation and Indoor Air to support and respond to incidents or sites containing radiological hazards. These teams provide expertise in radiation monitoring, radionuclide analyses, radiation health physics, and risk assessment.

REGIONAL RESPONSE TEAMS (RRT's) – Regional counterparts to the National Response Team, the RRT's comprise regional representatives of the Federal agencies on the NRT and representatives of each State within the region. The RRT's serve as planning and preparedness bodies before a response, and provide coordination and advice to the Federal OSC during response actions.

REGIONAL RESPONSE COORDINATION CENTERS (RRCC) – A standing facility operated by DHS/EPR/FEMA that is activated to coordinate regional response efforts, establish Federal priorities, and implement local Federal program support until a JFO is established in the field and/or the PFO, FCO or FRC can assume their NRP coordination responsibilities.

REPORTING LOCATION – Any one of six facilities/locations where incident assigned resources may check-in. The locations are: Incident Command Post-Resources Unit, Base, Staging Area, Helibase, or Division/Group Supervisors (for direct line assignments). Check-in occurs at one location only.

RESOURCES – All personnel and major items of equipment available, or potentially available, for assignment to incident tasks on which status is maintained.

RESPONDER REHABILITATION – Also known as "rehab", a treatment of incident personnel who are suffering from the effects of strenuous work and/or extreme conditions.

SAR ON-SCENE COORDINATOR (SAR OSC) – The SAR OSC coordinates the SAR mission on-scene using the resources made available by SMC and should safely carry out the SAR Action Plan. The SAR OSC may serve as a Branch Director or Group Supervisor to manage on-scene operations after the SAR mission is concluded and other missions continue, such as search and recovery.

SECTION – That organization level having functional responsibility for primary segments of an incident such as: Operations, Planning, Logistics and Finance. The Section level is organizationally between Branch and Incident Commander.

SENIOR FEDERAL OFFICIAL (SFO) – A SFO is an individual representing a Federal department or agency with primary statutory responsibility for incident management.

SINGLE RESOURCE – Is an individual, a piece of equipment and its personnel complement, or a crew or team of individuals with an identified work supervisor that can be used on an incident.

SITE SAFETY AND HEALTH PLAN (SSHP) – Site-specific document required by state and Federal OSHA regulations and specified in the Area Contingency Plan. The SSHP, at minimum, addresses, includes, or contains the following elements: health and safety hazard analysis for each site task or operation, comprehensive operations work plan, personnel training requirements, PPE selection criteria, site-specific occupational medical monitoring requirements, air monitoring plan, site control measures, confined space entry procedures (if needed), pre-entry briefings (tailgate meetings, initial and as needed), pre-operations commencement health and safety briefing for all incident participants, and quality assurance of SSHP effectiveness.

SITUATION ASSESSMENT – The evaluation and interpretation of information gathered from a variety of sources (including weather information and forecasts, computerized models, GIS data mapping, remote sensing sources, ground surveys, etc.) that, when communicated to emergency managers and decision makers, can provide a basis for incident management decision making.

SPAN OF CONTROL – A Command and Control term that means how many organizational elements may be directly managed by one person. Span of Control may vary from one to seven, and a ratio of five reporting elements is optimum.

STAGING AREA – That location where incident personnel and equipment are assigned awaiting tactical assignment. Staging Areas are managed by the OSC.

STAKEHOLDERS – Any person, group, or organization affected by and having a vested interest in the incident and/or the response operation.

STRATEGIC GOALS – Strategic goals are broad, general statements of intent.

STRATEGY – The general plan or direction selected to accomplish incident objectives.

STRATEGIC PLAN – Is a plan that addresses long-term issues such as impact of weather forecasts, time–phased resource requirements, and problems such as permanent housing for displaced disaster victims, environmental pollution, and infrastructure restoration.

STRIKE TEAM – Are specified combinations of the **same kind and type** of resources with common communications and a leader.

SUPERVISOR – ICS title for individuals responsible for command of a Division or Group.

SUPPORT ZONE – In a hazardous substance response, the clean area outside of the Contamination Control Line is a support zone. Equipment and personnel are not expected to become contaminated in this area. Special protective clothing is not required. This is the area where resources are assembled to support the hazardous substances/materials release operation.

SUPERVISOR OF SALVAGE AND DIVING (SUPSALV) – A salvage, search, and recovery operation established by the Department of Navy with experience to support response activities, including specialized salvage, firefighting, and petroleum, oil, and lubricants offloading.

TACTICAL DIRECTION – Directions given by the OSC that includes: the tactics appropriate for the selected strategy, the selection and assignment of resources, tactics implementation, and performance monitoring for each operational period.

TACTICS – Deploying and directing resources during an incident to accomplish the objectives designated by strategy.

TASK FORCE – A group of resources with common communications and a leader assembled for a specific mission.

T-CARD – Cards filled out with essential information for each resource they represent. The cards are color-coded to represent different types of resources.

TECHNICAL SPECIALISTS (THSP) – Personnel with special skills who can be used anywhere within the ICS organization.

TEMPORARY FLIGHT RESTRICTIONS (TFR) –TFRs are established by the Federal Aviation Administration (FAA) to ensure aircraft safety in the vicinity of the incident which restricts the operation of non-essential aircraft in the airspace around that incident.

TERRORISM – Any activity that: (1) involves an act that (a) is dangerous to human life or potentially destructive of critical infrastructure or key resources and (b) is a violation of the criminal laws of the United States or of any State or other subdivision of the United States; and (2) appears to be intended (a) to intimidate or coerce a civilian population, (b) to influence the policy of a government by intimidation or coercion, or (c) to affect the conduct of a government by mass destruction, assassination, or kidnapping.

UNACCEPTABLE RISK – Level of risk as determined by the risk management process which cannot be mitigated to an acceptable safe level.

UNIFIED COMMAND (UC) – An application of ICS used when there is more than one agency with incident jurisdiction or when incidents cross political jurisdictions. Agencies work together through the designated members of the Unified Command to establish their designated Incident Commanders at a single ICP and to establish a common set of objectives and strategies and a single Incident Action Plan. This is accomplished without losing or abdicating authority, responsibility, or accountability.

UNIFIED AREA COMMAND (UAC) – A unified area command is established when incidents under an area command are multi-jurisdictional.

UNIT – That organizational element having functional responsibility for a specific incident planning, logistics, or finance/administration activity.

VESSEL OWNER (VO) – VO is the owner/operator of the vessel or source which precipitated the incident.

VOLUNTEER – Any individual accepted to perform services by an agency that has authority to accept volunteer services when the individual performs services without promise, expectation, or receipt of compensation for services performed.

WATERSHED REHABILITATION – Is also known as "rehab"; restoration of watershed to as-near-as-possible its pre-incident condition, or to a condition where it can recover on its own.

WEAPON OF MASS DESTRUCTION (WMD) – As defined in Title 18, U.S.C. § 2332a: (1) any explosive, incendiary, or poison gas, bomb, grenade, rocket having a propellant charge of more than 4 ounces, or missile having an explosive or incendiary charge of more than one-quarter ounce, or mine or similar device; (2) any weapon that is designed or intended to cause death or serious bodily injury through the release, dissemination, or impact of toxic or poisonous chemicals or their precursors; (3) any weapon involving a disease organism; or (4) any weapon that is designed to release radiation or radioactivity at a level dangerous to human life.

ACRONYMS

AC	Area Command
A/C	Aircraft
ACO	Aircraft or Fixed-Wind Coordinator
ACP	Area Contingency Plan
ADCON	Administrative Control
AMS	Area Maritime Security
AMSC	Area Maritime Security Committee
AMSP	Area Maritime Security Plan
AMIO	Alien Migrant Interdiction Operations
AMVER	Automated Mutual-Assistance Vessel Rescue
AOBD	Air Operations Branch Director
AOIC	Assistant Officer In Charge
APSO	Asylum Pre-Screening Officer (INS)
ARC	American Red Cross
AREP	Agency Representative
ART	Alternate Response Technologies
ASGS	Air Support Group Supervisor
ATMWU	Air Transportable Mobile Weather Unit
ATOI	Air Target of Interest
ATC	Air Traffic Control
ATGS	Air Tactical Group Supervisor
BCMG	Base Manager
BO	Boarding Officer
BTM	Boarding Team Member
C2	Command and Control
C3	Command, Control, and Communications
CANUS	Canadian United States Joint Marine Pollution Contingency Plan
CAP	Civil Air Patrol
CASP	Computer-Assisted Search Planning
CASPER	C-130 Airborne Surveillance with Palletized Electronic Reconnaissance

25-27

CBDR	Constant Bearing, Decreasing Range
CBP	U.S. Customs and Border Protection
CC	Contributing Command
CCL	Contamination Control Line
CD	Counter Drug
CHET	Customs High Endurance Tracker (Cheyenne III aircraft)
CIC	Combat Information Center
CJCS	Chairman of the Joint Chiefs of Staff
CLMS	Claims Specialist
CO	Commanding Officer
COML	Communication Unit Leader
COMP	Compensation /Claims Unit Leader
COST	Cost Unit Leader
COTP	Captain of the Port
CRA	Coordinating Review Authority
CRC	Contamination Reduction Corridor
CRWD	Crew Boss/Crew Supervisor
CRZ	Contamination Reduction Zone
CSC	Combat Support Center
CTF	Commander Task Force
CTU	Commander Task Unit
D&M	Detention and Monitoring
DAN	Divers Alert Network
DCM	Dangerous Cargo Manifest
DEA	Drug Enforcement Administration
DFM	Diesel Fuel Marine
DHHS	Department of Health & Human Services
DHS	Department of Homeland Security
DIVS	Division/Group Supervisor
DMB	Datum Marker Buoy
DMOB	Demobilization Unit Leader
DOCL	Documentation Unit Leader
DOD	Department of Defense
DOT	Department of Transportation
DOSC	Deputy Operations Section Chief

DPIC	Deputy Incident Commander
DPRO	Display Processor
EEI	Essential Elements of Information
EEZ	Exclusive Economic Zone
ELT	Emergency Locator Transmitter
EMCON	Emission Control
EMS	Emergency Medical Services
EMT	Emergency Medical Technician
ENSP	Environmental Specialist
EOC	Emergency Operations Center
EOP	Emergency Operations Plan
EPA	Environmental Protection Agency, US
EPIC	El Paso Intelligence Center
EPIRB	Emergency Position Indicating Radio Beacon
EQPM	Equipment Manager
EQTR	Equipment Time Recorder
ERT	Emergency Response Team
ES	Electronic Surveillance
ESF	Emergency Support Functions
EUL	Environmental Unit Leader
EXCOM	Extended Communication Search
FAA	Federal Aviation Administration
FACL	Facilities Unit Leader
FC	Federal Coordinator
FDUL	Food Unit Leader
FEMA	Federal Emergency Management Agency
FLIR	Forward-Looking Infrared
FMSC	Federal Maritime Security Coordinator
FO	Facility Owner
FOB	Field Observer
FOD	Foreign Object Damage
FOG	Field Operations Guide
FOSC	Federal On-Scene Coordinator
FSC	Finance/Administration Section Chief

F/V	Fishing Vessel
GIS	Geographic Information System
GMDSS	Global Maritime Distress and Safety System
GSUL	Ground Support Unit Leader
H/C	Historic/Cultural
HAZ CAT	Hazardous Categorization Test
HAZMAT	Hazardous Materials
HAZSUB	Hazardous Substances
HCO	Helicopter Coordinator
HF	High Frequency
HLSA	Homeland Security Act
HSAS	Homeland Security Advisory System
HSPD-5	Homeland Security Presidential Directive No. 5
HSPD-7	Homeland Security Presidential Directive No. 7
HSPD-8	Homeland Security Presidential Directive No. 8
IAP	Incident Action Plan
IC	Incident Commander
ICE	U.S. Immigration and Customs Enforcement
ICP	Incident Command Post
ICS	Incident Command System
IECO	Immigration Emergency Coordinating Officer
IG	Immune Globulin
IMAT	Incident Management Assist Team
INCM	Incident Dispatcher
INJR	Compensation for Injury Specialist
INS	Incident of National Significance
IR	Infrared
ISB	In-situ Burn

JFO	Joint Field Office
JIC	Joint Information Center
JIS	Joint Information System
JRCC	Joint (aeronautical and maritime) Rescue Coordination Center
JRSC	Joint Rescue Sub-center
KIAS	Knots Indicated Air Speed
KT	Knot(s)
LCPL	Landing Craft Personnel, Large
LCU	Landing Craft, Utility
LE	Law Enforcement
LEA	Law Enforcement Agency
LEDET	Law Enforcement Detachment (USCG)
LEL	Lower Explosive Limit
LEU	Law Enforcement Unit
LKP	Last Known Position
LLLTV	Low Light Level Television
LNO	Liaison Officer
LPOC	Last Port of Call
LSC	Logistics Section Chief
M/V	Motor Vessel
MAC	Multi-agency Coordination
MARSEC	Maritime Security
MEDEVAC	Medical Evacuation
MEDICO	Medical Advice, Usually By Radio
MEDL	Medical Unit Leader
MEXUS	Mexican United States Joint Marine Pollution Contingency Plan
MINIRAD	Minimum Radiation
MLB	Motor Lifeboat
MLE	Maritime Law Enforcement
MOA	Memorandum of Agreement
MOOTW	Military Operations Other Than War

25-31

GLOSSARY & ACRONYMS   GLOSSARY & ACRONYMS

MOU	Memorandum of Understanding
MPA	Maritime Patrol Craft
MRCC	Maritime Rescue Coordination Center
MSST	Maritime Safety and Security Team
MTS	Marine Transportation System
MTSL	Marine Transportation System Recovery Unit
NCP	National Oil and Hazardous Substances Pollution Contingency Plan (40 CFR 300)
NDP	Naval Doctrine Publication
NIC	NIMS Integration Center
NIIMS	National Interagency Incident Management System
NIMS	National Incident Management System
NM	Nautical Mile
NMMSS	Naval Mast Mounted Sight System
NOAA	National Oceanic and Atmospheric Administration
NOTAM	Notice to Airmen
NPFC	National Pollution Funds Center
NPOC	Next Port of Call
NRC	National Response Center (Phone number (800)424-8802)
NRP	National Response Plan
NRDAR	Natural Resource Damage Assessment
NRS	National Response System
NSSE	National Special Security Event
NTSB	National Transportation Safety Board
NVD	Night Vision Devices
NVG	Night Vision Goggles
NWP	Naval Warfare Publication
OC	Oleoresin Capsicum (Pepper Spray)
OCC	Operations Coordination Center
OIC	Officer-In-Charge

OPA 90	Oil Pollution Act of 1990
OPBD	Operations Branch Director
OPCEN	USCG Operations Center
OPCON	Operational Control
OPLAN	Operation Plan
OPORDER	Operation Order
OPSEC	Operations Security
ORDM	Ordering Manager
O/S	On-Scene
OSC	Operations Section Chief
OSC	SAR On-Scene Coordinator
OSHA	Occupational Safety and Health Administration
P/C	Pleasure Craft
PA	Programmatic Agreement (Historical/Cultural Protection)
PD-27	Presidential Directive 27
PDW	Personal Defense Weapon
PFD	Personal Flotation Device
PIO	Public Information Officer
PIW	Person(s) in Water
PML	Personal Marker Light
POB	Persons On Board
POC	Point-of-Contact
POD	Probability of Detection
POS	Probability of Success
PPE	Personal Protective Equipment
PQS	Personnel Qualification Standard
PRA	Primary Review Authority
PRECOM	Preliminary Communication Search
PRFA	Pollution Removal Funding Authorization
PROC	Procurement Unit Leader
PSC	Planning Section Chief
PTRC	Personnel Time Recorder
PWCS	Ports, Waterways and Coastal Security

QI	Qualified Individual
QRT	Quick Reaction Team
R&A	Rescue and Assistance
RAR	Resources at Risk
RB-M	Response Boat - Medium
RB-S	Response Boat - Small
RBDF	Royal Bahamian Defense Force
RCC	Rescue Coordination Center
RCP	Regional Response Plan
RCDM	Receiving and Distribution Manager
RDD	Radiological Dispersal Device
REHB	Responder Rehabilitation Manager
RESL	Resource Unit Leader
RIB/RHIB	Rigid Hull Inflatable Boat
RIT	Rapid Intervention Team
ROE	Rules of Engagement
RRBT	Rapid Response Boarding Team
RRD	Radiological Dispersion Devise
RRT	Regional Response Team
RSC	Rescue Sub-Center
SAR	Search and Rescue
SART	Search and Rescue Transponder
SARTEL	SAR Telephone (private hotline)
SATCOM	Satellite Communications
SC	SAR Coordinator
SCAT	Shoreline Cleanup Assessment Team
SCKN	Status/Check-In Recorder
SECM	Security Manager
SEHS	Special Event Homeland Security
SELEX	Selected Exercise
SITL	Situation Unit Leader
SLAR	Side Looking Airborne Radar
SLDMB	Self-Locating Datum Marker Buoy
SMC	SAR Mission Coordinator
SNO	Statement of No Objection

SOFR	Safety Officer
SOLAS	Safety of Life at Sea
SONS	Spill of National Significance
SOSC	State On-Scene Coordinator
SPUL	Supply Unit Leader
SRA	Safe Refuge Area
SRB	Surf Rescue Boat
SRIE	Safety Rules of Engagement
SROE	Standing Rules of Engagement
SRR	Search and Rescue Region
SRU	Search Rescue Unit
SS	Expanding Square Search
SSI	Sensitive Security Information
SSC	Scientific Support Coordinator
SSHP	Site Safety and Health Plan
STAM	Staging Area Manager
STVE	Strike Team Leader, Vessel
SUBD	Support Branch Director
SURPIC	Surface Picture
S/V	Sailing Vessel
SVBD	Service Branch Director
T/V	Tank Vessel
TACLET	Tactical Law Enforcement Team
TACON	Tactical Control
TB	Tuberculosis
TDS	Time, Distance and Shielding
TFLD	Task Force Leader
TFR	Temporary Flight Restrictions
THC	Tetrahydrocannibanol
THSP	Technical Specialist
TIME	Time Unit Leader
TOI	Target of Interest
TRACEM	Thermal, Radioactive, Asphyxiation, Chemical, Etiological, and Mechanical
TSA	Transportation Security Administration
TSI	Transportation Security Incident

TTP	Tactics, Techniques, and Procedures
UAC	Unified Area Command
UC	Unified Command
UHF	Ultra-High Frequency
UMIB	Urgent Marine Information Broadcast
USC	United States Code
USCG	United States Coast Guard
USMC	United States Marine Corps
USN	United States Navy
UTL	Utility Boat
VERTREP	Vertical Replenishment
VESS	Vessel Support Unit Leader
VHF	Very High Frequency
VO	Vessel Owner
VS	Sector Search
WTD	Water-Tight Door